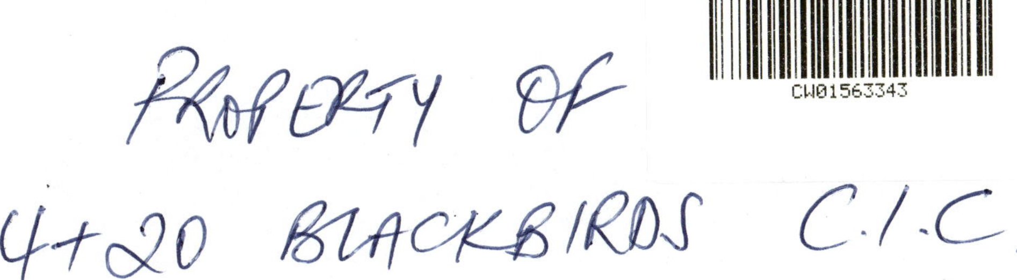

Royal cookery: or, the complete court-cook Containing the choicest receipts in all the particular branches of cookery, now in use in the Queen's palaces By Patrick Lamb, To which are added, bills of fare for every season in the year

Patrick Lamb

Royal cookery; or, the complete court-cook. Containing the choicest receipts in all the particular branches of cookery, now in use in the Queen's palaces ... By Patrick Lamb, ... To which are added, bills of fare for every season in the year.
Lamb, Patrick
ESTCID: T091554
Reproduction from Harvard University Houghton Library
Another issue bears the imprint: printed for Maurice Atkins. With a half-title, and two final leaves of advertisements.
London : printed for Abel Roper, and sold by John Morphew, 1710.
[16],127,[17]p.,plates ; 8°

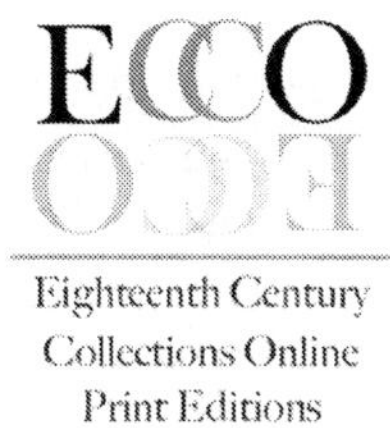

Gale ECCO Print Editions

Relive history with *Eighteenth Century Collections Online*, now available in print for the independent historian and collector. This series includes the most significant English-language and foreign-language works printed in Great Britain during the eighteenth century, and is organized in seven different subject areas including literature and language; medicine, science, and technology; and religion and philosophy. The collection also includes thousands of important works from the Americas.

The eighteenth century has been called "The Age of Enlightenment." It was a period of rapid advance in print culture and publishing, in world exploration, and in the rapid growth of science and technology – all of which had a profound impact on the political and cultural landscape. At the end of the century the American Revolution, French Revolution and Industrial Revolution, perhaps three of the most significant events in modern history, set in motion developments that eventually dominated world political, economic, and social life.

In a groundbreaking effort, Gale initiated a revolution of its own: digitization of epic proportions to preserve these invaluable works in the largest online archive of its kind. Contributions from major world libraries constitute over 175,000 original printed works. Scanned images of the actual pages, rather than transcriptions, recreate the works ***as they first appeared.***

Now for the first time, these high-quality digital scans of original works are available via print-on-demand, making them readily accessible to libraries, students, independent scholars, and readers of all ages.

For our initial release we have created seven robust collections to form one the world's most comprehensive catalogs of 18th century works.

Initial Gale ECCO Print Editions collections include:

> ***History and Geography***
> Rich in titles on English life and social history, this collection spans the world as it was known to eighteenth-century historians and explorers. Titles include a wealth of travel accounts and diaries, histories of nations from throughout the world, and maps and charts of a world that was still being discovered. Students of the War of American Independence will find fascinating accounts from the British side of conflict.

Social Science

Delve into what it was like to live during the eighteenth century by reading the first-hand accounts of everyday people, including city dwellers and farmers, businessmen and bankers, artisans and merchants, artists and their patrons, politicians and their constituents. Original texts make the American, French, and Industrial revolutions vividly contemporary.

Medicine, Science and Technology

Medical theory and practice of the 1700s developed rapidly, as is evidenced by the extensive collection, which includes descriptions of diseases, their conditions, and treatments. Books on science and technology, agriculture, military technology, natural philosophy, even cookbooks, are all contained here.

Literature and Language

Western literary study flows out of eighteenth-century works by Alexander Pope, Daniel Defoe, Henry Fielding, Frances Burney, Denis Diderot, Johann Gottfried Herder, Johann Wolfgang von Goethe, and others. Experience the birth of the modern novel, or compare the development of language using dictionaries and grammar discourses.

Religion and Philosophy

The Age of Enlightenment profoundly enriched religious and philosophical understanding and continues to influence present-day thinking. Works collected here include masterpieces by David Hume, Immanuel Kant, and Jean-Jacques Rousseau, as well as religious sermons and moral debates on the issues of the day, such as the slave trade. The Age of Reason saw conflict between Protestantism and Catholicism transformed into one between faith and logic -- a debate that continues in the twenty-first century.

Law and Reference

This collection reveals the history of English common law and Empire law in a vastly changing world of British expansion. Dominating the legal field is the *Commentaries of the Law of England* by Sir William Blackstone, which first appeared in 1765. Reference works such as almanacs and catalogues continue to educate us by revealing the day-to-day workings of society.

Fine Arts

The eighteenth-century fascination with Greek and Roman antiquity followed the systematic excavation of the ruins at Pompeii and Herculaneum in southern Italy; and after 1750 a neoclassical style dominated all artistic fields. The titles here trace developments in mostly English-language works on painting, sculpture, architecture, music, theater, and other disciplines. Instructional works on musical instruments, catalogs of art objects, comic operas, and more are also included.

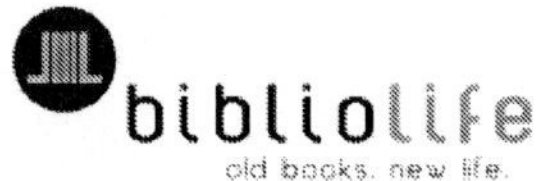
biblioLife
old books. new life.

Royal Cookery; or, the Complete Court-Cook.

CONTAINING THE

Choiceſt Receipts

In all the particular Branches of

COOKERY,

Now in Uſe in the QUEEN'S

PALACES

OF

St. *James's*, *Kenſington*, } *Hampton-Court*, and *Windſor.*

With near Forty Figures (curiouſly engraven on *Copper*) of the magnificent Entertainments at *Coronations*, *Inſtalment*, *Balls*, *Weddings*, &c. at Court; Alſo Receipts for making the *Soupes*, *Jellies*, *Biſques*, *Ragoo's*, *Pattys*, *Tanzies*, *Forc'd-Meats*, *Cakes*, *Puddings*, &c.

By PATRICK LAMB, *Eſq*;
Near 50 Years Maſter-Cook to their late Majeſties King *Charles* II. King *James* II. King *William* and Queen *Mary*, and to Her Preſent Majeſty Queen *ANNE*.

To which are added,
Bills of Fare for every Seaſon in the Year

London, Printed for *Abel Roper*, and ſold by *John Morphew*, near *Stationers-Hall.* 1710.

THE PREFACE.

WEre there no other Reaſon for a Preface *to this* Treatiſe, *the very Subject of it ſeems to beſpeak one: For as it conſiſts of a Sett of Entertainments as nice and delicate as any Court or Country can boaſt of; ſo is it common in the caſe of Treats, beſides the* Preface *of an Invitation, to diſpoſe the Gueſts into their ſeveral Places, and ſometimes to prepare their Appetites, by giving 'em, beforehand, a ſhort* Bill *of* Fare. *In Compliance with which laudable Cuſtom, I hope, I may be allow'd, as far at leaſt as the Parallel will bear, to take my* Readers *by the Hand, and introduce them with ſome* Decency *to this viſionary Treat; eſpecially, ſince every Gueſt is like to pay his Shot, before he has any Title to the* Banquet. *How far, at laſt, it will anſwer the Expence either of his Purſe or Patience, he muſt judge for himſelf, after he has taſted the ſeveral Diſhes; only let him conſider, that ſuch Feaſts come, like Swallows, but once in a Seaſon, and then perhaps he may not grudge either his Pains or his Penny: As for thoſe ſeverer Aſceticks who keep* Lent *at* Chriſtmas, *and weigh out their* Diet *by Drams and Scruples, it muſt not be expected they ſhould purchaſe a Piece with ſo hungry a Title to it, as thinking, perhaps, that Luxury will thrive faſt enough without ſtudy'd Receipts to ſeaſon and recommend it. But as a vicious Palate is, by no means, a proper Judge of Taſtes, ſo were it a*

great

great Pity, One or Two peevish Cynicks should put Good-Eating out of Countenance; especially, since the Author *has not here undertaken to* cook *out an Art of* Gluttony, *or to teach the Rich and Lazy, how to grow fatter, by ranging* Epicurism *under the several Heads of* Jellies, Soupes, *and* Pottages; *but his chief Aim was to represent the* Grandeur *of the* English *Court and Nation, by an Instance which lay most within his View and Province; the Magnificence, I mean, of those publick* Regales *made on the more solemn Occasions of admitting Princes to their* Thrones, *Peers to their* Honours, *Ambassadors to their* Audience, *and Persons of Figure to the* Nuptial-Bed. *Now, these are Solemnities which call for good Looks and better* Chear *than ordinary; what in other Cases might be justly term'd* Profuseness, *does, in this, change its*

Name, and become a Debt, both to Cuſtom and Decency: And, in Truth, no Kingdom in the World either deſerves, or has acquir'd a better Name, on the ſcore of a frank and hoſpitable Genius, than this of Great-Britain; *for as the Soil itſelf has bleſs'd us with an amazing Plenty; ſo has God likewiſe bleſs'd us with an Openneſs of Spirit to diffuſe and ſcatter it, to all around us, inſomuch that in the Space of Four ſucceeding Reigns, the City of* London, *and the* Royal Palaces, *have furniſh'd out more noble and ſumptuous Entertainments, than, perhaps,* Rome *ſaw Triumphs during the Time of her* Cæſars: *Not that there lies any juſt Compariſon between Solemnities of ſo different a kind; but if we take in the Courſes of the one, as well as the other, (among which our glorious Victories have not wanted their Share) I do not ſee why theſe* Feſtivities *may not*

claim

claim a Place in our Annals, *as well as the Ovations of the Old* Romans; *Nay, perhaps, the Advantage may lay on our Side, when 'tis consider'd, that they slew the Sheep purely in Compliment to their* Gods, *but we in Honour to our Country, and in Charity to our Neighbours, the best Effects, surely, of our Gratitude to Heaven. Besides which, I may venture to say, that our Credit and Esteem with Foreign Ministers, has, in a great Measure, been built and supported on this Foundation; For, those whose Shortness of Parts, or, perhaps, Residence among us, would not qualify 'em to remark upon the nicer Part of our Constitution, have yet gone away with such a* Relish *of our Magnificence, as to lament their own Barrenness, whenever they reflected on the* Flesh-Pots *they left behind them. For the Want of which substantial and wholsome Plenty, the* Quelque Chose

of

of France, *and the Vines of* Italy *make no better Amends, than the* Surfeits *and* Fevers *they usually bring on such as deal in them. --- As for the Author of these Sheets, his Name and Character are so well known and establish'd in all the Courts of* Christendom, *that I need observe no more of him, than that he liv'd and dy'd a very great Rarity, having maintain'd his Station at Court, and the Favour of his Prince, for about Fifty Years together; which whoever does after him, may boast of being one of the Two fortunate and long-liv'd Courtiers, which perhaps an Hundred Ages before have not produc'd.*

CON-

CONTENTS.

Forc'd

CONTENTS.

Plum

CONTENTS.

Orange

CONTENTS.

The

The Contents of the Tables; *with Directions for the* Book-binders *where to place them.*

Plate

Royal

Royal Cookery:

OR, THE

COMPLETE
COURT-COOK.

To make Soupe-Santé.

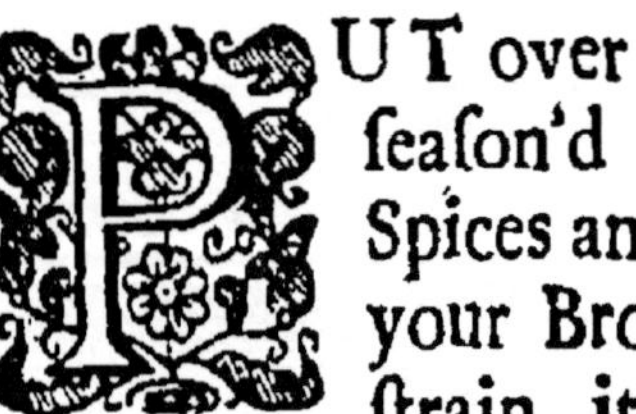

UT over 12 Pound of Beef, ſeaſon'd moderately with Spices and Salt; boil it till your Broth is ſtrong, and ſtrain it out to a good Knuckle of Veal blanch'd; then boil it up a ſecond Time, putting your Pullet to it that you deſign to put in the Mid-

A dle

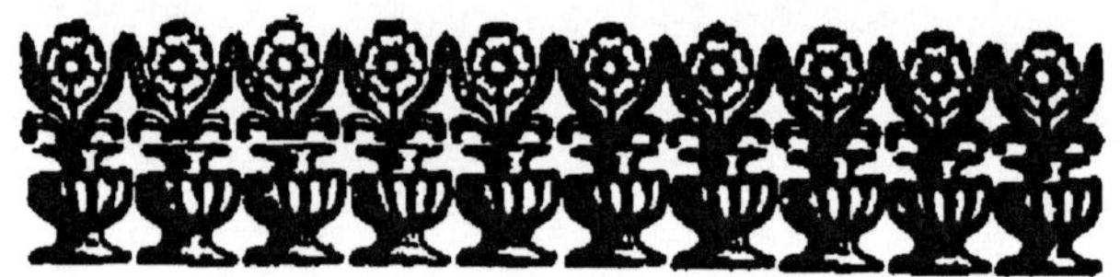

Royal Cookery:

OR, THE

COMPLETE *COURT-COOK.*

To make Soupe-Santé.

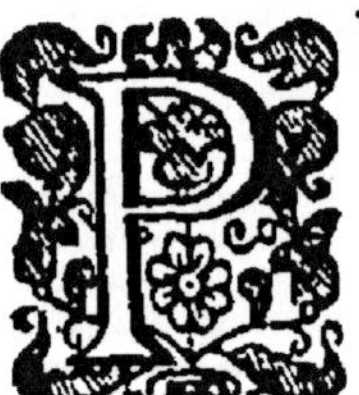

PUT over 12 Pound of Beef, seaſon'd moderately with Spices and Salt; boil it till your Broth is ſtrong, and ſtrain it out to a good Knuckle of Veal blanch'd; then boil it up a ſecond Time, putting your Pullet to it that you deſign to put in the Middle of your Soupe; let it boil till it comes to the Strength of a Jelly; put to it in the boiling a Bit of Bacon, that is not rusty, stuck with Six Cloves. Your Broth being thus ready, at the same time, make a Pan of good Gravy, thus. Take a Stew-pan or Brass-dish, place in the Bottom of it a Quarter of a Pound of Bacon, cut in Slices, clean from Rust, likewise the Bigness of half an Egg of Butter; Take 5 or 6 Pound of a Fillet of Veal, and cut it in Slices, twice as thick as you do for Scotch Collops, and place on your Bacon in your Stew-pan, covering all the Bottom over If you have no Veal, use Buttock-Beef. Set it over a clear Fire, not very hot, and let it colour by degrees. Give it an Hour and a Half to colour. When it begins to crack, put a little of the Fat of your boiling Broth to it; stir it as little as possible because it makes it thick, and throw in 3 or 4 slic'd Onions, one Carrot, two Turneps, a little Parsley, a Sprig of Thyme, a little whole Pepper, and Cloves. All these Ingredients being fry'd together till you think it comes to a good Colour, if in Summer, a few Mushrooms will give it a good Taste.

Being

Being of a good Colour, add to your boiling Broth from your Knuckle of Veal aforesaid, leaving some to keep your Veal and Pullet white, to soak your Bread with it for your Soupe, and other Uses in the Kitchen Your Broth and Gravy being in Readiness, take such Herbs as the Country where you are will afford; such as Sallary, Endive, Sorrel, a little Chervil or Cabbage-Lettice well pick'd and wash'd; mince them down with your Mincing-Knife, and squeeze the Water from them, and place them in a little Pot, or deep Saucepan; put to them so much of your Broth and Gravy, as will just cover them; let them boil tender; then take the Crust of two *French* Rolls, and boil up with 3 Pints of Gravy, and strain it thro' a Strainer or Sieve, and put it to your Herbs: If you have no *French* Bread to thicken it with, take the Bigness of an Egg of Butter, a small Handful of Flower, and brown it over the Fire, and a little minc'd Onion, if the Eaters be Lovers of it; if not, let the Onion that was in your Gravy serve. Add to your Brown some Gravy, and boil it, and strain it thro' a Sieve to your

Herbs, instead of your *French* Bread aforesaid. Let your Herbs be pretty tender, before you put your Thickning in: Boil all together half an Hour, and skim off the Fat. Place in the Bottom of your Dish that you intend to serve your Soupe in, some *French* Bread in Slices, or the Crust dry'd before the Fire, or in an Oven; boil it up with some of your Broth; so put your Fowl and Herbs on the Top of it. Let your Garnishing be a Rim on the Outside of it, tender boil'd, Sallary or Endive boil'd in good Broth, and cut in Pieces about three Inches long; if you cannot spare Herbs, take a Bit of Forc'd Meat and boil'd Carrot to garnish *So serve it hot.* Take care there is no Fat on it. This is a Summer, or a Winter Soupe, where you can have Herbs. And this is the *French* Fashion of *Soupe-Santé*.

Queens Dinner. February 6. 1704.

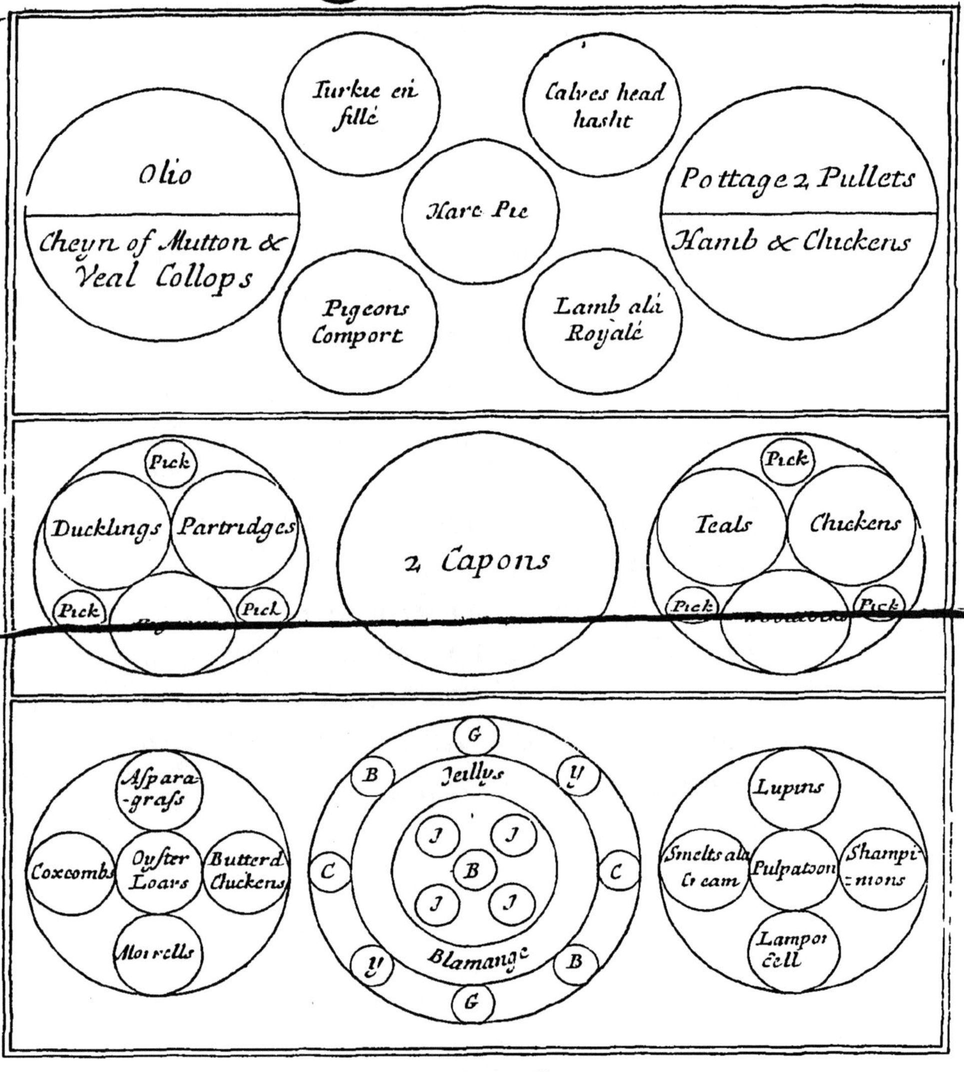

Olio

Cheyn of Mutton & Veal Collops

Turkie en fillé

Calves head hasht

Hare Pie

Pigeons Comport

Lamb alá Royalé

Pottage 2 Pullets

Hamb & Chickens

Pick

Ducklings

Partridges

Pick

[illegible]

Pick

2 Capons

Pick

Teals

Chickens

Pick

[illegible]

Pick

Asparagrass

Coxcombs

Oyster Loavs

Butterd Chickens

Moirells

G

B

Jellys

Y

C

J

J

B

J

J

C

Y

Blamange

B

G

Lupins

Smelts ala Cream

Pulpatoon

Shampinions

Lampor Eell

Middle Dishes

2 of Lupins	2 of Blamange	2 of Coxcombs
2 of Oysters	2 of Yellow	2 of Srimps
2 of Sweetbreads	2 of Crystal	2 of Larks
2 of Asparagrass	2 of [illegible]	[illegible]

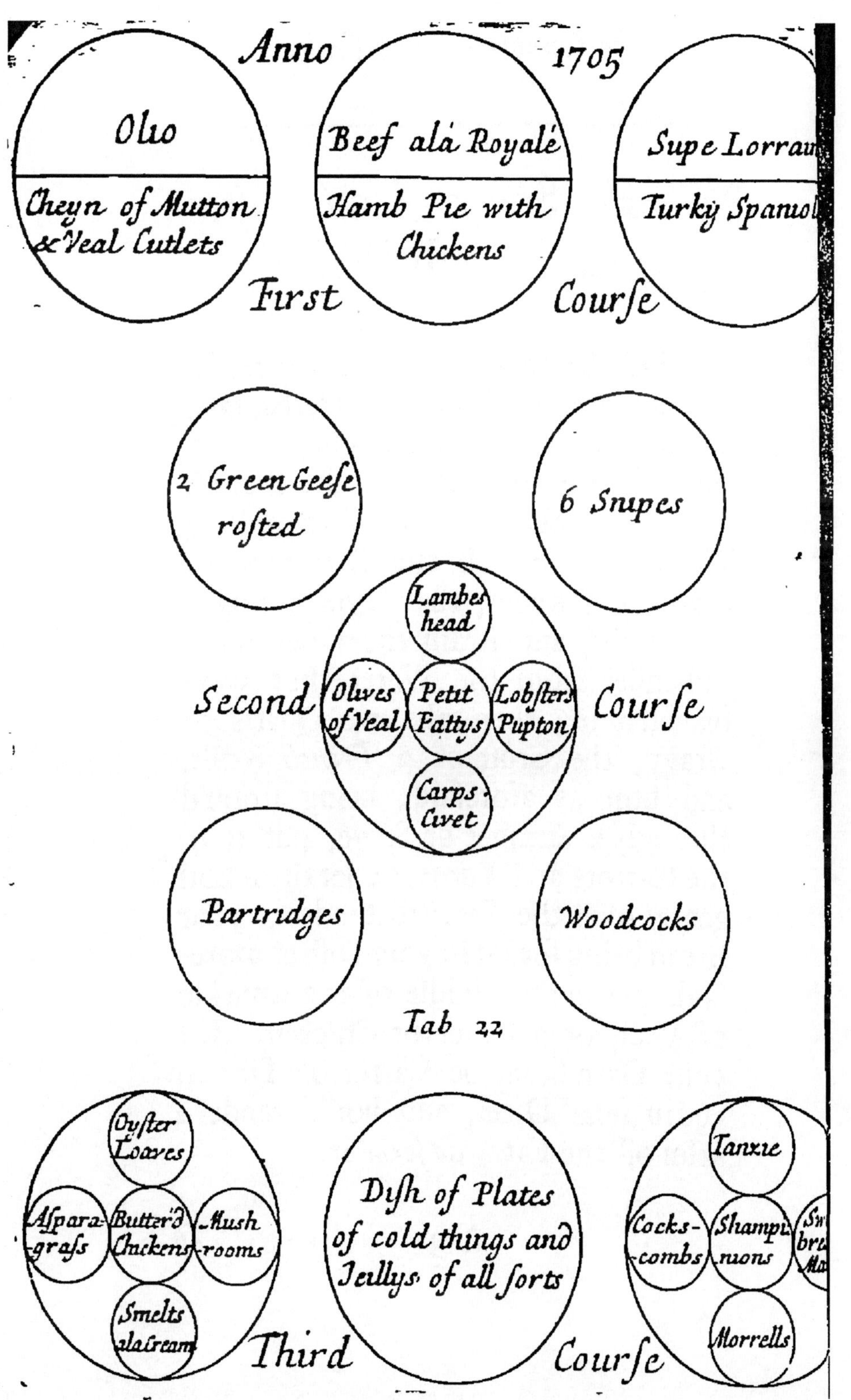
Anno 1705
Olio
Cheyn of Mutton
& Veal Cutlets
Beef alá Royalé
Hamb Pie with
Chickens
Supe Lorrai
Turky Spaniol
First Course
2 Green Geese
rosted
6 Snipes
Lambes
head
Second
Olives
of Veal
Petit
Pattys
Lobsters
Pupton
Course
Carps
Civet
Partridges
Woodcocks
Tab 22
Oyster
Loaves
Aspara-
-grass
Butter'd
Chickens
Mush
-rooms
Smelts
alaCream
Third
Dish of Plates
of cold things and
Jellys of all sorts
Course
Tanxie
Cocks-
-combs
Shampi-
-nions
Morrells

To make Soupe-Santé, *after the* Engliſh *Way.*

YOUR Broth and Gravy being ready as aforeſaid, inſtead of Herbs, take Carrots and Turneps, and cut them in Slices ſquare, an Inch long, the Bigneſs of a Quill; blanch them off in boiling Water, but blanch the Carrots more than the Turneps, the Turneps only 2 or 3 Boils, and ſtrain them out on a Cullender from the Water they were blanch'd in; then take two Quarts of Gravy, the Cruſt of 2 *French* Rolls, and boil as aforeſaid, being ſtrain'd through a Strainer or Sieve, put it to the Carrots and Turneps; let them boil gently over the Fire till tender; your Bread being ſoak'd in your Diſh as aforeſaid, put in the Middle of it a Knuckle of Veal, or a Pullet or Chicken. Let your Garniſhing be Carrot or Turnep cut in ſmall Dices, and boil'd tender; skim off the Fat. *So ſerve it.*

To make Malgré-Santé.

PRovide your Herbs as aforesaid for your *French Soupe Santé*; if it is not for *Catholicks*, put to them Broth, boil them tender, and put to them a Brown of Flower prepar'd as aforesaid: Let your Garnishing be Carrot and Turneps, in the Middle a *French* Roll fry'd, with the Crum taken out at the Bottom, soak your Bread in Broth, and put your Herbs over it. *So serve it.* If your Master will have no Broth, you must use Water, or Water from boil'd Pease. In this Case, you must fry your Herbs in Butter and a little Onion; be sure take the Fat off, when you add your Pease, Broth, or boiling Water. *So serve it.*

To make a White Malgré-Soupe.

TAKE 6 Heads of Endive, a Handful of Sorrel, a little Chervil, Parſley, and Onion, minc'd ſmall, and Herbs minc'd alſo, being very clean waſh'd, ſtew them down in a Sauce-pan, with a Quarter of a Pound of Butter, for a Quarter of an Hour; then add 2 Quarts of clear Broth, or boiling Water, if the Maſter will have no Broth. Your Herbs being boil'd tender, skim the Fat off, and thicken your Herbs with the Yolks of 10 or 12 Eggs, according to the Bigneſs of your Diſh; ſcrape a Nutmeg, and the Juice of half a Lemon, if your Sorrel is not ſharp enough. Your Bread being ſoak'd in your Diſh as aforeſaid, put in the Middle of it a *French* Roll fry'd. Let your Garniſhing be 8 or 10 poach'd Eggs, and fry'd Bread betwixt 'em, on the Outſide of your Rim on the Diſh, cut in ſmall Dice; you may put a poach'd Egg on the Top of your *French* Roll in the Middle of your Soupe, being juſt thicken'd up with your Eggs hot over the Fire. Set off your Diſh on the Table, before you fill it up, becauſe your Eggs may not curdle in your Soupe. *So ſerve it.*

To make Peaſe, *or* Purée-Soupe; *as the* French *call it.*

HAving good Broth, made of Veal, Fowl, and Beef, as I told you in the firſt Receipt; If in Summer, take Green Peaſe; if they be very young, give them but a little Boil in Water, ſtrain 'em out, and pound them in a Mortar; make a Cowley in a Sauce-pan with the Things following. A Quarter of a Pound of Butter, Half a Quarter of a Pound of Bacon cut in ſmall Dices, 2 Onions ſlic'd a Sprig of Thyme, a little Parſley, the Cruſt of a *French* Roll, a little whole Pepper and Cloves; Fry all theſe over the Fire, gently

gently, till your Bread is pretty crisp, but take care you burn not your Herbs. This being done, add to it two or three Quarts of Broth, according to the Quantity of your Pease, and Bigness of your Dish; so boil it up, and skim the Fat off, before you put in your beaten Pease; then mix your Pease in your Cowley over the Fire, and let them boil up together, so strain them thro' a Strainer or Sieve; this being done, and your Bread soak'd in your Dish as aforesaid, you may put in the Middle of your Dish a Duck or Ducklings, a Green Goose, or Pigeons, or a Knuckle of Veal. Let your Garnishing be Cucumers split, and the Cores taken out, boil'd tender in good Broth, round your Rim of Paste or Forc'd Meat. If your Pease be very young, you may put a few whole ones in your strain'd *Purée*, being tender boil'd first in Water or small Broth. *So serve it.* In the Winter time, you may take Blue Pease, and boil them first tender in Water, and then strain them out from it, and put them into your Cowley of Broth and Ingredients as aforesaid, only colouring it with a little Juice of Spinnage, instead of Green Pease.

Peaſe; in your ſtrain'd *Purée,* you may uſe the Tops of Aſparagus, cut in Bits tender boil'd. Your Garniſhing, Aſparagus; you may ſtew a little Sorrel in this *Purée.* *So ſerve it.*

To make Soupe-Borſwoy.

HAving good Broth and Gravy in Readineſs, take Four Bunches of Sallary, and 10 Heads of Endive, being clean waſh'd, and the Outſide taken off; cut them in Pieces Inch long, ſwing them well from the Water. This Soupe may be made Brown or White: If you intend it Brown, put your Herbs into 2 Quarts of boiling Gravy, being firſt blanch'd in boiling Water 5 or 6 Minutes; Then take the Cruſt of 2 *French* Rolls, boil it up in 3 Pints of Gravy, ſtrain it thro' a Strainer or Sieve, and put it to the Herbs, when they are almoſt ready; For that is to be minded in all Soupes, that your Thickning is not to be put in, till your Herbs are almoſt tender: You may put in the Middle

dle of your Soupe a Pullet or Chickens. Your Garniſhing a Rim, and on the Outſide ſome of your Sallary cut in Pieces 3 Inches long, your Bread being ſoak'd in ſome good Broth or Gravy, and your Herbs boiling hot. *So ſerve it.*

To make Soupe-Borſwoy *in the Spring, when there is no* Sallary *nor* Endive.

TAKE 12 Cabbage-Lettice, 6 Green Cucumers, pare them and take the Cores out, cut both Cucumers and Lettice in little Bits about Inch long, ſcald 'em off in boiling Water, and put them to clear, ſtrong Broth; let 'em boil tender with a Handful of Green Peaſe. The Fowl that you intend to put in the Middle of your Soupe, you may boil with your Herbs; skim the Fat off, boil your Bread in ſome of the ſame Broth. Let your Garniſhing be Cucumers and Lettice. Uſe no Thickning in this Soupe. *So ſerve it.*

To

To make a Turnep-Soupe.

HAving good Veal-Gravy in Readineſs, take ſome good Turneps, pare them and cut them in Dices, 1 or 2 Dozen, according to their Bigneſs, and the Bigneſs of your Diſh; fry them of a brown Colour in clarify'd Butter or Hogs Lard. Take two Quarts of good Gravy, and the Cruſts of two *French* Rolls, boil'd up together and ſtrain'd thro' a fine Strainer. Your Turneps being ſtrain'd from the Fat they were fry'd in; put them together, boil them till tender. You may roaſt a Duck to put in the Middle. Let your Garniſhing be a Rim, on the Outſide of it ſome ſmall dic'd Turneps boil'd white in Broth, and betwixt every Parcel of them, a Piece of fry'd Turnep, in Shape of a Cock's Comb. Soak your Bread in ſome good Fat and Gravy, take them up. *And ſo ſerve it.*

To

To make a Soupe *of* Savoy *or* Cabbage.

LET your Savoys be cut in four Pieces, and 3 Parts boil'd in fair Water; then ſqueeze them, when cold, with your Hand, clean from the Water; place them into a large Sauce-pan or little Braſs Diſh, ſuch a Quantity as your Diſh will hold: There muſt be Room betwixt each Piece of Savoy to take up Soupe with a large Spoon. Put them a boiling with as much Broth or Gravy as will cover them. Set them Stewing over the Fire 2 Hours before Dinner. At the ſame time, take a Sauce-pan with a Quarter of a Pound of Butter, put it over the Fire with a Handful of Flower, keep it ſtirring till brown; put to it two minc'd Onions, and ſtir it a little afterwards; then put to it a Quart of Veal-Gravy, boil it a little, and pour all over your Savoys as afore-ſaid. You may force Pigeons betwixt the Skin and the Body with good Forc'd Meat, made of Veal; or you may take a Duck or Ducklings, being truſs'd up for boiling; then fry them off, and put 'em Stewing with your Savoys. Let a little Bacon, ſtuck with Cloves, be put in with them to ſtew. Garniſhing be a Rim, and on the Outſide of it Slices of Bacon, a little Savoy betwixt each Slice. Taking the Fat clean off, ſoak your Bread in your Diſh, with ſome good Broth or Gravy; ſo place your Savoys at a due Diſtance, and your Fowl in the Middle. *So ſerve it.*

To make Soupe Vermiſelly.

TAke 2 Quarts of good Broth made of Veal and Fowl, put to it about Half a Quarter of a Pound of Vermiſelly, a Bit of Bacon ſtuck with Cloves; take the Bigneſs of Half an Egg of Butter, and rub it together with Half a Spoonful of Flower, and diſſolve it in a little Broth to thicken your Soupe: Boil a Pullet or Chickens for the Middle of your Soupe. Let your Garniſhing be a Rim, on the Outſide of it Cut Lemon, ſoak your Bread in your Diſh with ſome of the ſame Broth. Take

the

Kings Dinner at my Lord Ranelaughs

May 20 1700

First Course

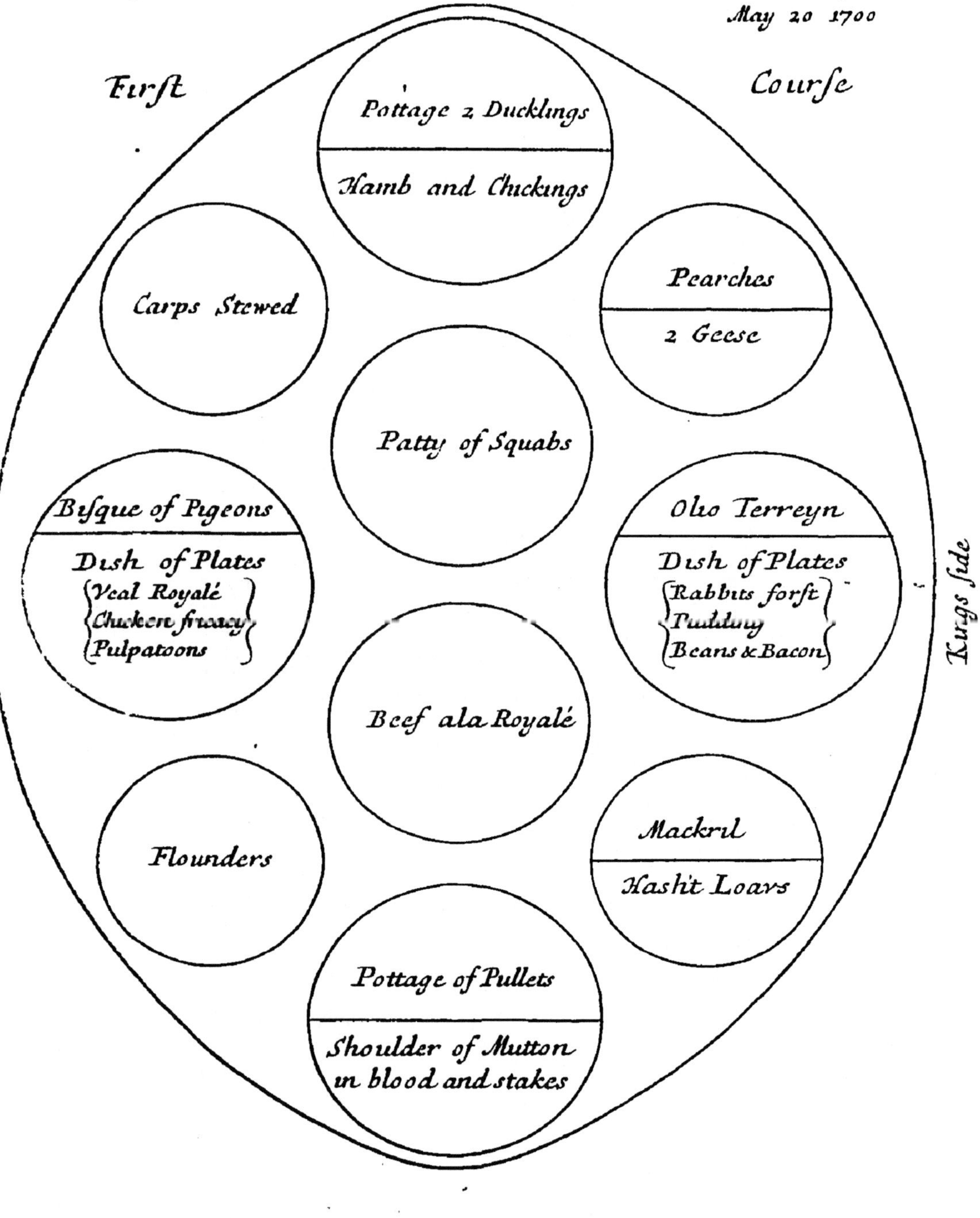

Pottage 2 Ducklings

Hamb and Chickings

Carps Stewed

Pearches

2 Geese

Patty of Squabs

Bisque of Pigeons

Dish of Plates
- Veal Royalé
- Chicken fricacy
- Pulpatoons

Olio Terreyn

Dish of Plates
- Rabbits forst
- Pudding
- Beans & Bacon

Kings side

Beef ala Royalé

Flounders

Mackril

Hash't Loavs

Pottage of Pullets

Shoulder of Mutton in blood and stakes

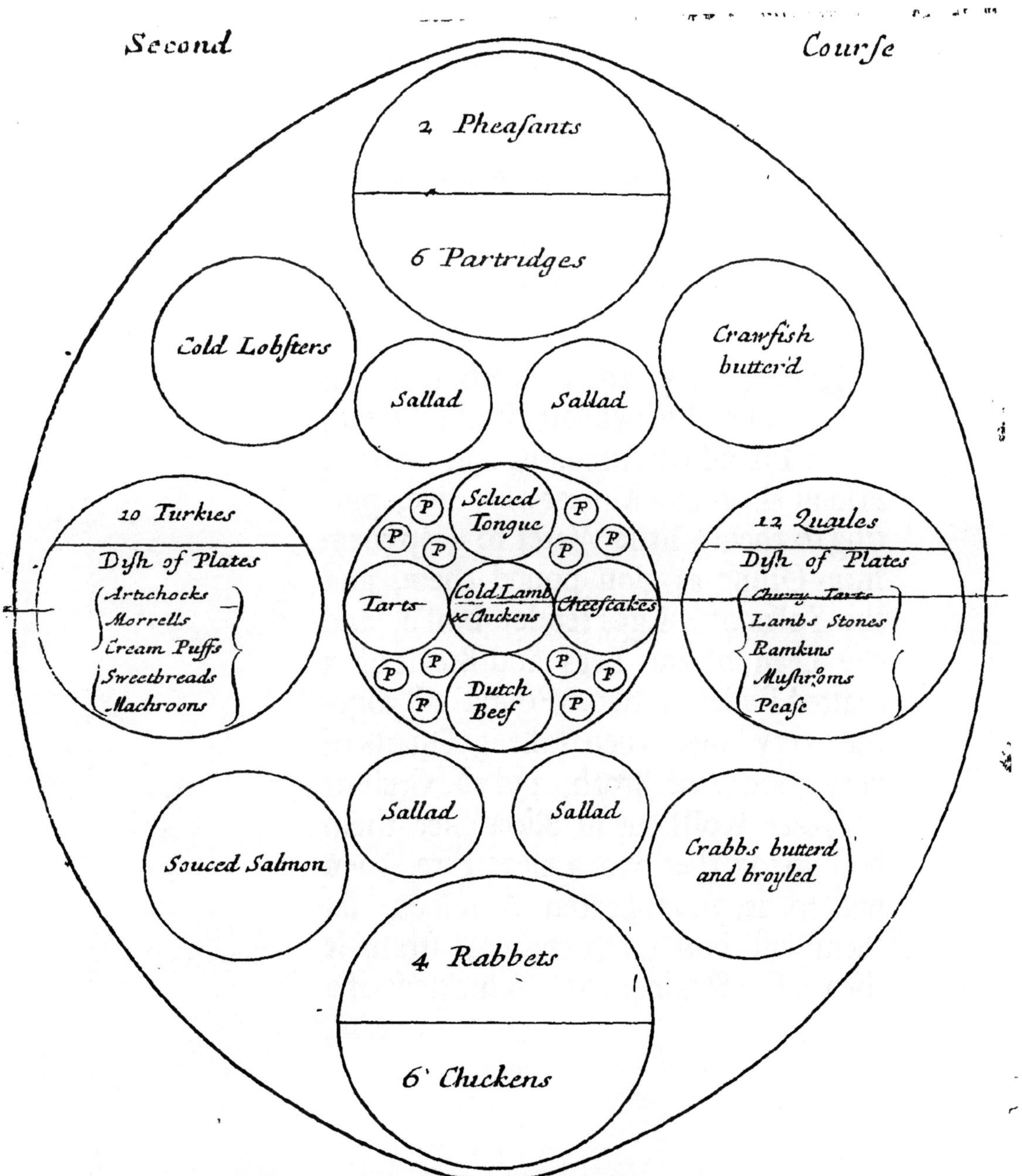
Second
Course
2 Pheasants
6 Partridges
Cold Lobsters
Sallad
Sallad
Crawfish butter'd
10 Turkies
Dish of Plates
Artichocks
Morrells
Cream Puffs
Sweetbreads
Machroons
Scliced Tongue
Tarts
Cold Lamb & Chickens
Cheesecakes
Dutch Beef
P
12 Quailes
Dish of Plates
Cherry Tarts
Lambs Stones
Ramkins
Mushroms
Pease
Sallad
Sallad
Souced Salmon
Crabbs butterd and broyled
4 Rabbets
6 Chickens

the Fat off, and put your Vermiſelly in your Diſh. *So ſerve it.* You may make a Rice-Soupe the ſame Way, only your Rice being firſt boil'd tender in Water, and it muſt boil an Hour in ſtrong Broth. Whereas, Vermiſelly but half an Hour.

To make Soupe-Lorrainé.

HAving very good Broth made of Veal and Fowl, and ſtrain'd clean, take a Pound of Almonds, and blanch; Pound them in a Mortar very fine, putting to them a little Water to keep them from Oiling as you pound them, and the Yolks of 4 Eggs tender boil'd, and the Lean of the Legs and Breaſt of a roaſted Pullet or two. Pound all together very fine; then take 3 Quarts of very good Veal Broth, and the Cruſt of 2 *French* Rolls cut in Slices; let them boil up together over a clear Fire, then put to it your beaten Almonds, let them juſt boil up together, ſtrain it thro' a fine Strainer to the Thickneſs of a Cream, the Fat off, and put your Vermiſelly in your Diſh. *So ſerve it.* You may make a Rice-Soupe the ſame Way, only your Rice being firſt boil'd tender in Water, and it muſt boil an Hour in ſtrong Broth. Whereas, Vermiſelly but half an Hour.

To make Soupe-Lorrainé.

HAving very good Broth made of Veal and Fowl, and ſtrain'd clean, take a Pound of Almonds, and blanch; Pound them in a Mortar very fine, putting to them a little Water to keep them from Oiling as you pound them, and the Yolks of 4 Eggs tender boil'd, and the Lean of the Legs and Breaſt of a roaſted Pullet or two. Pound all together very fine; then take 3 Quarts of very good Veal Broth, and the Cruſt of 2 *French* Rolls cut in Slices; let them boil up together over a clear Fire, then put to it your beaten Almonds, let them juſt boil up together, ſtrain it thro' a fine Strainer to the Thickneſs of a Cream,

Cream, as much as will ſerve the Bigneſs of your Diſh; mince the Breaſts of 2 roaſted Pullets, and put them into a Loaf as big as 2 *French* Rolls, the Top cut off, and the Crum cut out; ſeaſon your Haſh with a little Pepper and Salt, ſcrape a Nutmeg, and the Bigneſs of an Egg of Butter, five or ſix Spoonfuls of your ſtrain'd Almonds: The Bread that you put in the Bottom of your Soupe, let it be *French* Bread dry'd before the Fire, or in an Oven. So ſoak it with clear Broth, and a little of your ſtrain'd Soupe; Place your Loaf in the Middle, put in your Haſh warm; you may put 4 Sweetbreads, tender boil'd, about your Loaf, if you pleaſe. Let your Garniſhing be a Rim, and ſlic'd Lemon *So ſerve it.*

To make Crawfish *or* Lobster-Soupe.

YOUR Crawfish or Lobster-Soupe being boil'd: If Crawfish, pick the Shells off of the Tail of 'em, and leave the Bodies, Tails, and Legs together, the Quantity of two Dozen, to garnish your Dish: If your Dish is large, you ought to have a hundred Crawfish. Pick the Tails out of the rest from the Shells; put them in a Sawce-pan; then you'll find a little Bag at the End next the Claws, which is bitter like Gall, that you must take care to throw away; likewise you must throw away any thing that is white and woolly in the Belly. Then put the Shells in a marble or wooden Mortar, and pound them to a Paste. While your Shells are thus pounding, put in a large Sawce-pan or

Stew-pan, three Quarters of a Pound of Butter, the Cruſt of two *French* Rolls, three or four Onions, ſlic'd, two Dozen Corns of whole Pepper, one Dozen of Cloves, a Sprig of Thyme, a Handful of Parſley; fry theſe Ingredients ſoftly over the Fire half a Quarter of an Hour, till your Bread is criſp, but take care you do not burn your Herbs. At the ſame time, take care to prepare your Fiſh for your Stock, which is to be two Carps, two Eels, and a Thornback; if you cannot have Carp, you muſt uſe Whitings or Flounders, in the place of Carp, with your Eel and Thornback; skin the Carps and Eels, and cut the thick Fiſh from the Back of your Carp, and ſave it to make a Forc'd Meat of: And likewiſe ſave the Head and Bones of your Carp as you can, in order to be forc'd in the Middle of your Soupe. Then chop your Eel to Pieces, and skin'd Thornback or what other freſh Fiſh you have, four or five Pound Weight; and put them to your aforeſaid Ingredients, ſtewing over the Fire, and let them ſtew half an Hour together, ſtirring them now

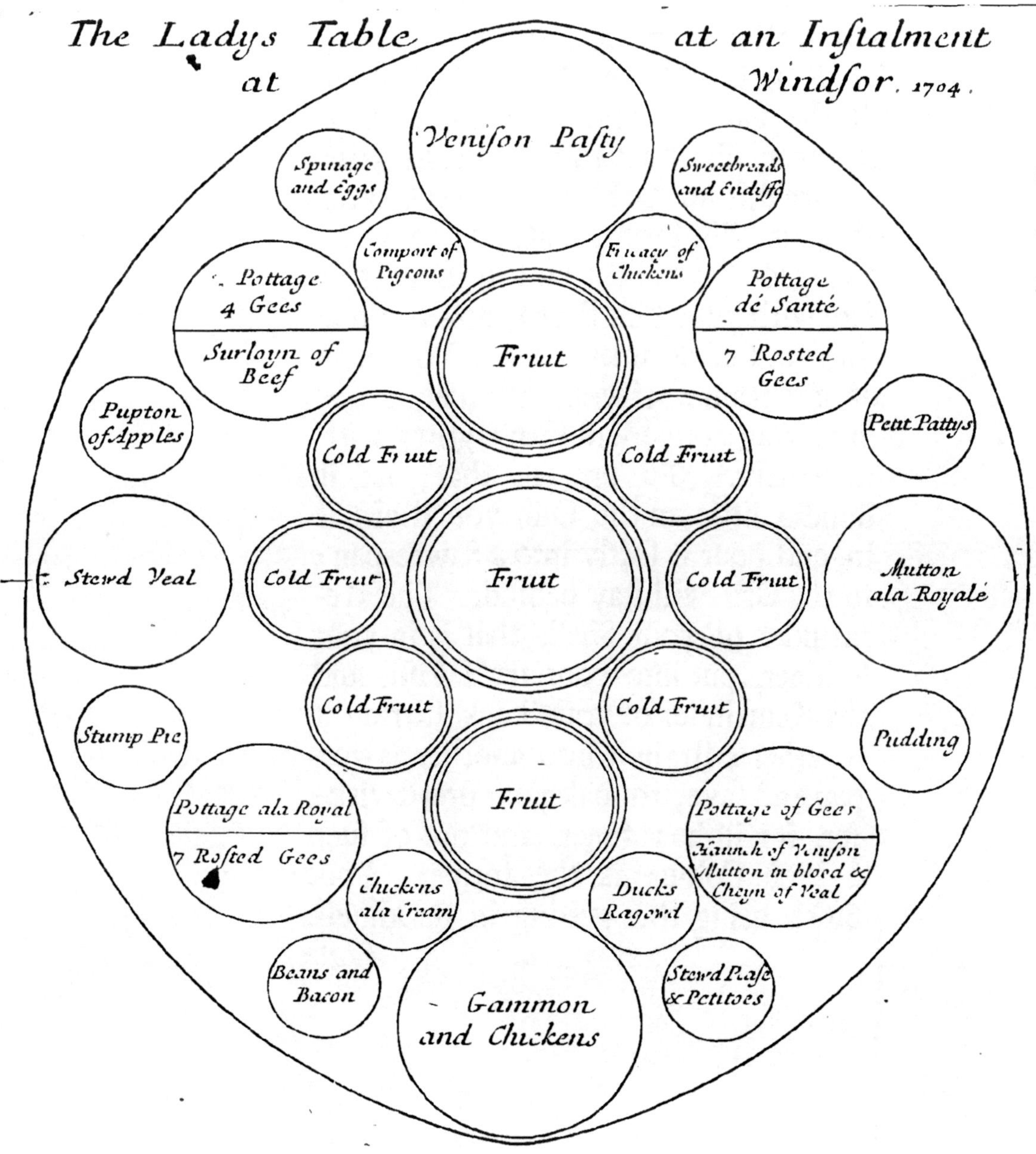

The Ladys Table at an Instalment at Windsor. 1704.
Venison Pasty
Spinage and Eggs
Sweetbreads and Endiffe
Comport of Pigeons
Fricacy of Chickens
Pottage 4 Gees
Surloyn of Beef
Pottage de Santé
7 Rosted Gees
Fruit
Pupton of Apples
Petit Pattys
Cold Fruit
Cold Fruit
Stewd Veal
Cold Fruit
Fruit
Cold Fruit
Mutton ala Royale
Cold Fruit
Cold Fruit
Stump Pie
Pudding
Pottage ala Royal
7 Rosted Gees
Fruit
Pottage of Gees
Haunch of Venison Mutton in blood & Cheyn of Veal
Chickens ala Cream
Ducks Ragowd
Beans and Bacon
Gammon and Chickens
Stewd Plase & Petitoes

now and then, that they burn not to the Bottom. When the Rawneſs is fry'd off of the Fiſh, then pour in four or five Quarts of boiling Water or Broth, and ſeaſon it moderately with Salt; let it boil half an Hour, then skim all the Fat off, and take up, with a Skimmer, all the Cruſt of Bread that was fry'd, from the Fiſh, and two Quarts of your Fiſh-Broth, and put to your pounded Crawfiſh; boil it over the Fire with your Fiſh-Broth, and ſtrain it thro' a fine Strainer, to the Thickneſs of a Cream: If your Strainer is not fine, your Soupe will prove gritty with the Shells. To prevent that, let it ſtand a little in the Diſh you ſtrain it in, and pour it ſoftly into a Sawce-pan; ſo the Grit will ſtay behind. The Remainder of your Shells that is in your Strainer, put into your fry'd Fiſh, and the Remainder of your Stock, ſtirring it together; ſtrain it into another Sawce-pan, and ſave, to ſoak your Bread with; for, it will be thinner, and not of ſuch a high Colour as the former. Your Stock being thus getting in Readineſs;

caufe the Fiſh that you cut off the Back of your Carp-Fiſh, to be minc'd fine, and add to it, three or four Butter'd Eggs, the Crum of a *French* Roll, boil'd in Milk or Cream, a boil'd Onion, and a little Parſley minc'd fine, the Bigneſs of an Egg of Butter, a little Pepper and Salt, ſcrape a Nutmeg, ſqueeze in half a Lemon: Mince all theſe together to a Paſte, then force the Bodies of your Carps, where you cut your Fiſh off into the ſame Shape as they were, ſmoothing them over with your Hand and a beaten Egg; pour over a little melted Butter, ſtrew it over a little Handful of grated Bread; then bake it three Quarters of an Hour, before you have Occaſion for it, buttering the Bottom of your Pan or Mazarine you bake it in. Let your Bread be cut in thin Slices, and dry'd before the Fire, or in an Oven, and ſoak'd in ſome of your thin Stock: Then take your Carps up from the Fat, and place it in the Middle of your Diſh; then put the Tails of your Crawfiſh that you pick'd formerly, into your beſt Stock; boil it up only over the Fire, be-

fore

fore you ſend it away, ſqueeze in half a Lemon, then pour it round your bak'd Carp in your Pottage-Diſh. Let your Garniſhing be a Rim of the ſame Forc'd Meat, or if it is ſcarce, take lean Paſte, and on the Outſide of it two Dozen of Crawfiſh, as was ſpoke of in the Beginning of the Receipt, being firſt hot in a little of your Stock. I would not have been ſo large in this Receipt; but you are to take Notice, to make the Stock for any other Fiſh-Soupe, the ſame as you do for this, and likewiſe the Forc'd Meat. All the Difference will be in the Middle, and the Garniſhing likewiſe in the Colour, for only Crawfiſh or Lobſter-Soupe can be of a red Colour. *So ſerve it.*

To make a Lobſter-Soupe.

LET a Forc'd Meat of Fiſh be made as aforeſaid, only in place of Carps, you may take Tench, Pike, Trout, or Whitings, and Flounders; or what other freſh Fiſh the Country where you are, can afford, to the Value of four or five Pound Weight. Make your Stock of it as aforeſaid, keep your Forc'd Meat as clean from Bones as poſſible as you can, and make it up in Bigneſs of a double *French* Roll, being hollow in the Middle, and open on the Top; bake it half an Hour before you uſe it, place it in the Middle of your Soupe. At the ſame time, let the Spawn of your Lobſters, being two or four of them, according to the Bigneſs of your Diſh; ſtrain it thro' with your Cowley, as you did your Crawfiſh-Soupe; And take the Meat

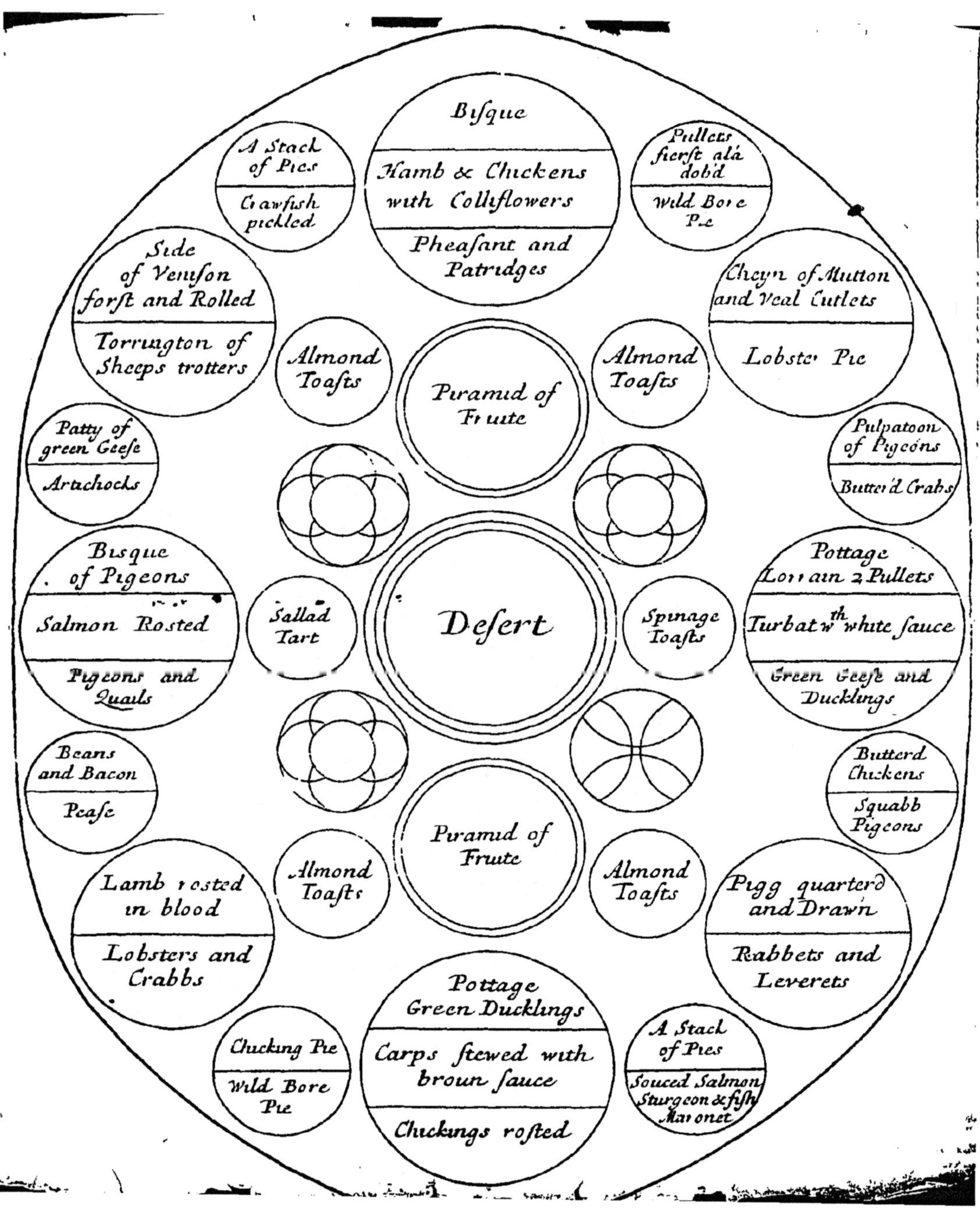

Bisque
Hamb & Chickens with Colliflowers
Pheasant and Patridges
A Stack of Pies
Crawfish pickled
Pullets fierst alá dob'd
Wild Bore Pie
Side of Venison forst and Rolled
Torrington of Sheeps trotters
Cheyn of Mutton and Veal Cutlets
Lobster Pie
Almond Toasts
Piramid of Fruite
Almond Toasts
Patty of green Geese
Artachocks
Pulpatoon of Pigeons
Butter'd Crabs
Bisque of Pigeons
Salmon Rosted
Pigeons and Quails
Sallad Tart
Desert
Spinage Toasts
Pottage Lorrain 2 Pullets
Turbat wth white sauce
Green Geese and Ducklings
Beans and Bacon
Pease
Butterd Chickens
Squabb Pigeons
Almond Toasts
Piramid of Fruite
Almond Toasts
Lamb rosted in blood
Lobsters and Crabbs
Pigg quarterd and Drawn
Rabbets and Leverets
Pottage Green Ducklings
Carps stewed with broun sauce
Chickings rosted
Chicking Pie
Wild Bore Pie
A Stack of Pies
Souced Salmon Sturgeon & fish Maronet

Meat of your Lobſters, and cut it in large Dice; warm it up in a Sawce-pan with a little of the Cowley, a little Pepper and Salt, ſqueeze a Lemon, a little Butter; put it in your Forc'd Loaf in the Middle of your Soupe. Your Bread being ſoak'd, and your Cowley hot, ſqueeze in a little Lemon; and diſh it up. Let your Garniſhing be a Rim of Paſte, the Outſide cut Lemon. *So ſerve it.*

To make a Muſcle-Soupe.

TAKE a Quantity of Muſcles, and make them clean, and boil them and pick them out of the Shells; put them in a Sawce-pan, waſh them clean after they are out of the Shells; then take three or four Pound of freſh Fiſh and a Cowley, as for the Crawfiſh-Soupe, and ſtrain it thro' to the Thickneſs of a Cream; put a little of it to your Muſcles; cut off the Top of a *French* Roll, take out the Crum, and fry it in a little Butter; place it in the Middle of your Soupe, your Bread being ſoak'd with ſome of your Cowley. Let your Garniſhing be a Rim of Paſte; lay the Muſcle-Shells round the Outſide of it; thicken up your Muſcles with the Yolk of an Egg, as you do a Fricaſſee, and put one or two in each Shell, round your Soupe; likewiſe fill up the Loaf in the Middle, the Cowley being boiling hot, ſqueeze into it, and the Muſcles, a little Lemon. *So ſerve it.* You may do a Cockle-Soupe the ſame Way.

To

To make a Scate *or* Thornback-Soupe.

MAKE your Stock or Cowley as you did for your Crawfish-Soupe, only you have no Shells to put in it for colouring your Scate or Thornback; being skin'd, take half a Pound of the best of the Fish from the Bones to Pieces, and throw into your Cowley, with some other fresh Fish as the Country affords. Your Cowley being strain'd off ready,as for your Crawfish-Soupe, to the Thickness of a Cream; mince the lean Part of the Fish you cut from the Bones, and put over the Fire in a little Sawce-pan with a little Butter, Pepper and Salt, stirring it till the Raw is off of it; then mince it with your Knife on a clean Table the second time,then put it in your Swace-pan again: If it is good Fish, it will

will eat as tender as a Chicken haſh'd; put a little Lemon to it, and put it in a *French* Roll in the Middle of your Soupe; your Cowley being hot, and your Bread ſoak'd in the Bottom of your Diſh, ſqueeze in ſome Lemon. Let your Garniſhing be a Rim on the Outſide. *So ſerve it.*

To make a Purée-Malgré.

PRovide your Peaſe, and every thing, as you did for your *Purée-Soupe*, only put in the Middle of your Soupe, inſtead of Fowl, a *French* Roll fry'd. Let your *Purée* be of a Cream Thickneſs. Garniſhing, a Rim of Paſte, and Lemon cut round it, your Bread being ſoak'd in your Diſh. *So ſerve it.*

My Lady Arrans Daughters Wedding Supper

June 6 1699.

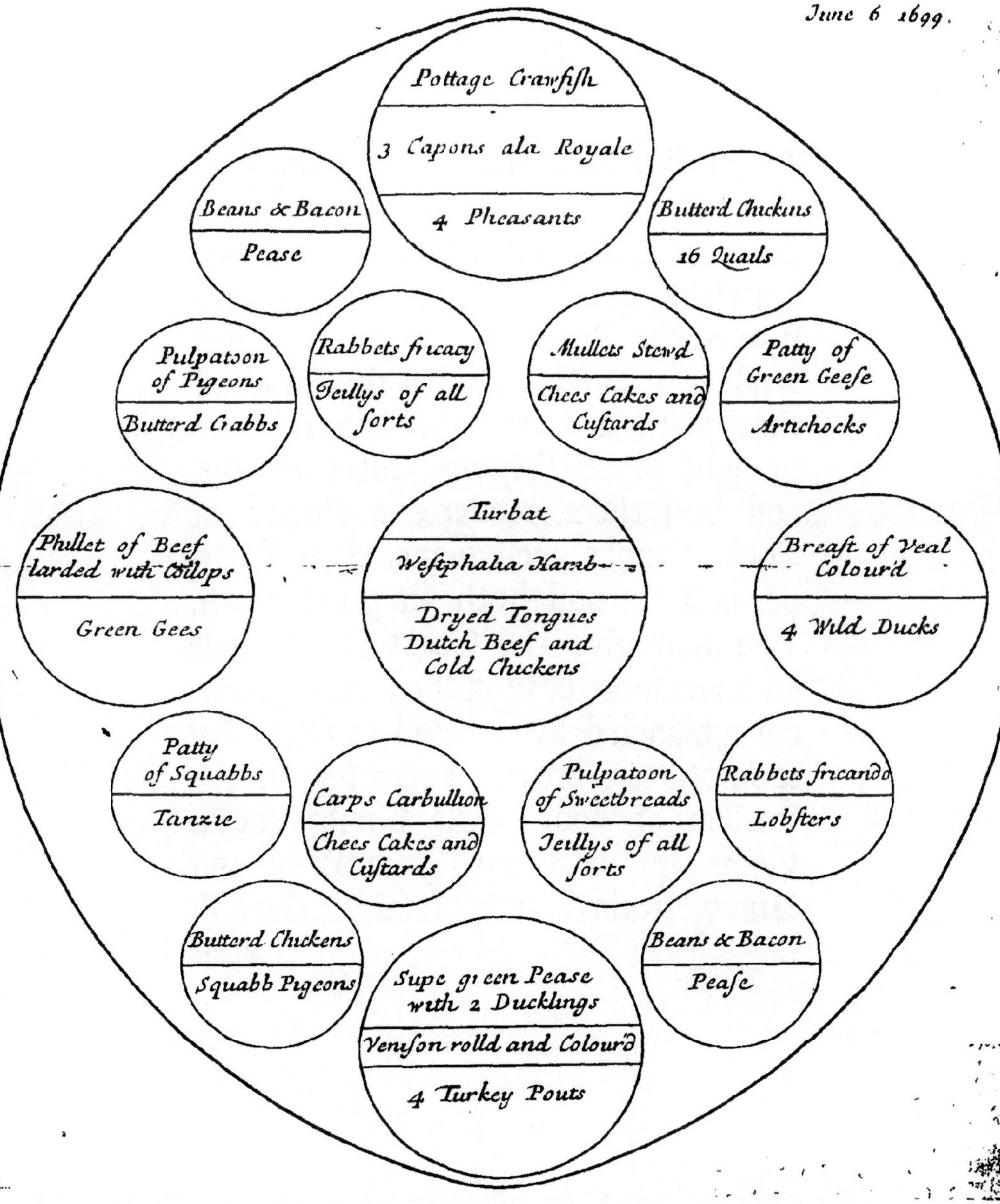

Pottage Crawfish
3 Capons ala Royale
4 Pheasants

Beans & Bacon
Pease

Butterd Chickins
16 Quails

Pulpatoon of Pigeons
Butterd Crabbs

Rabbets fricacy
Jellys of all sorts

Mullets Stewd
Chees Cakes and Custards

Patty of Green Geese
Artichocks

Phillet of Beef larded with Collops
Green Gees

Turbat
Westphalia Hamb
Dryed Tongues Dutch Beef and Cold Chickens

Breast of Veal Colour'd
4 Wild Ducks

Patty of Squabbs
Tanzie

Carps Carbullion
Chees Cakes and Custards

Pulpatoon of Sweetbreads
Jellys of all sorts

Rabbets fricando
Lobsters

Butterd Chickens
Squabb Pigeons

Supe green Pease with 2 Ducklings
Venison rolld and Colourd
4 Turkey Pouts

Beans & Bacon
Pease

To make a Biſque *of* Pigeons.

YOUR Broth and Gravy being prepar'd as for your *Soupe-Santé*, put the Cruſt of two *French* Rolls, with two Quarts of good Veal-Gravy, and boil it over the Fire, ſtrain it thro' a fine Strainer or Sieve, rubbing the Bread all thro' with a Laddle. Then take ſix or eight Squab-Pigeons, truſs them up, and boil them tender; a Pound of Cocks Combs well blanch'd and tender-boil'd; boil both in good Broth. You muſt give the Cocks Combs half an hours more boiling than the Pigeons; cut a blanch'd Sweetbread in Dice, fry it in Butter, brown, and a few of the ſmalleſt of your Cocks Combs cut in Pieces; put both into your Bread and Gravy, ſtrain'd as aforeſaid. Garniſh your

your Diſh with a Rim of Paſte, and the biggeſt of your Cocks Combs on the Outſide of it; your Bread being ſoak'd in your Diſh with good Broth and Gravy, place your Pigeons round in the Middle, and boil up your Cowley with the fry'd Sweetbreads and Cocks Combs. Let your Cowley be of a Cream Thickneſs, ſqueeze in half a Lemon. *So ſerve it.*

To make Soupe-Profitrollé.

HAving good Broth and Gravy as for your Biſque: If your Diſh is large, take four Partridges; if ſmall, two: If you have no Partridges, take two Pheaſants, roaſt them off; when roaſted, take the Lean of the Breaſts of one or two, make a Haſh of it; put it in the Middle of a *French* Roll, the Top taken off, the Crum taken out and fry'd; ſeaſon

ſeaſon your Haſh with a little Broth, a Bit of Butter, Pepper and Salt, ſcrape a Nutmeg, ſqueeze a Lemon; ſave the Breaſts cut from the Back of two of your Partridges whole, and take the Skin off of 'em, and two whole Sweetbreads; place the Loaf in the Middle of your Diſh with the Haſh, and the two Breaſts and two Sweetbreads plac'd over-againſt one another; put the Bones of your Partridges or Pheaſants in a Mortar and pound them, keeping out the Rumps, if they are ſtale, or taſte of the Green-Corn. Make your Cowley of a Quarter of a Pound of Butter, the Cruſts of two *French* Rolls, two Onions ſlic'd, a little whole Pepper and Cloves; fry all this gently over the Fire a Quarter of an Hour; then add to them, two Quarts of Veal-Gravy, boil it up, skim the Fat off; Put to it your pounded Bones, boil all up together and ſtrain it thro' a fine Strainer, rubbing it with your Ladle to the Thickneſs of a Cream; warm your Sweetbreads and Breaſts of Partridges in the ſame Cowley. Garniſhing, a Rim and Lemon; all things being

ing boiling hot, ſqueeze in a little Lemon in the Cowley. *So ſerve it.*

To make an Olio.

AT ſix a Clock in the Morning, put over a Leg of Beef, about ſix Pound of Brisket-Beef, cut in five or ſix Pieces, ſeaſon'd moderately with Spices and Salt; skim it, let it boil till your Broth is very ſtrong; take a Neck of Veal, a Neck of Mutton, a Piece of a Loin of Pork; if no Pork, then take half a Pig, or if you have neither of them, take half a Gang of Hog's Feet, boil them tender with good Seaſoning; Cut your Mutton, Pork, and Veal, in ſquare Pieces, two Ribs to a Piece, skin your Pork, give it all two or three Boils in boiling Water, then let it drain in a Cullender; when drain'd, either roaſt it or fry it of a good Colour; if you roaſt it, you muſt do it quick, that it

A Dinner at Esqr. Hills at Teddington

January 3 1707

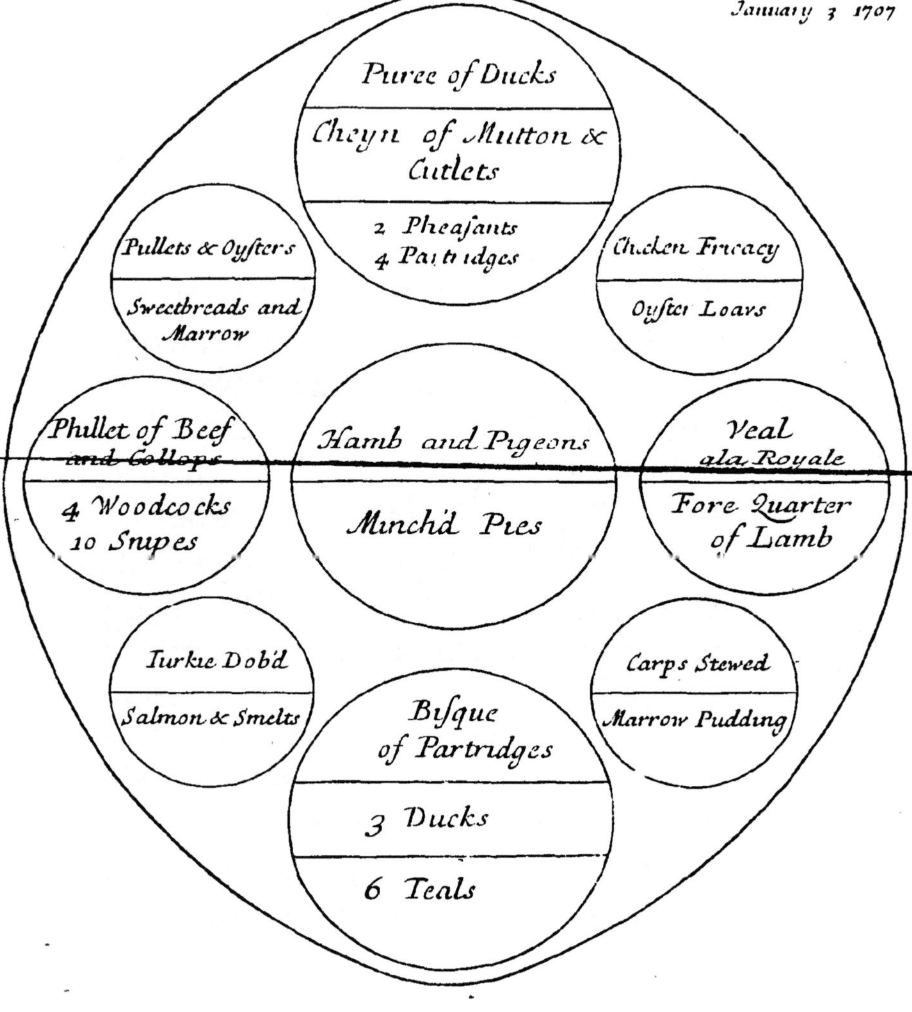

Puree of Ducks

Cheyn of Mutton & Cutlets

2 Pheasants
4 Partridges

Pullets & Oysters

Sweetbreads and Marrow

Chicken Fricacy

Oyster Loavs

Phillet of Beef and Collops

4 Woodcocks
10 Snipes

Hamb and Pigeons

Minch'd Pies

Veal ala Royale

Fore Quarter of Lamb

Turkie Dob'd

Salmon & Smelts

Carps Stewed

Marrow Pudding

Bisque of Partridges

3 Ducks

6 Teals

it loſe not its Gravy. Then take your Brisket-Beef out of your aforeſaid Broth, not being quite tender, becauſe it muſt boil along with the aforeſaid Meat; place it in a large Braſs Diſh or Stew-pan. At the ſame time, get ready the Roots and Herbs following; Three Savoys cut in four Pieces each, ſix Carrots cut in long Slices, two Parſneps cut in long Slices, two Bunches of Sallary, ſix Leek-heads Hand long, twelve Parſley Roots, ſix Heads of Endive or Cabbage-Lettice; Put over five or ſix Dozen of Carrots, Turneps, and Onions, the Bigneſs of Yolks of Eggs; blanch all theſe off in boiling Water, and drain them on a Cullender; Then tie each ſort of the Herbs up by itſelf, tying them with a Piece of Pack-Thread twice round; place it into your aforeſaid Stew-pan, with your aforeſaid Meat, and ſtrain your Broth from your Leg of Beef, thro' a Sieve, on the Top of your Meat and Herbs, as much as barely covers, and ſet it a boiling ſoftly three Hours before you uſe: Then fry off your Turneps, Carrots, and Onions,

that

that was cut round, in Hog's Lard or Clarify'd Butter; place them into a Sawce-pan; then get the Fowls following, or what the Country can afford, *viz.* Two Chickens, two Pigeons, two Woodcocks, four Snipes, two Teals or Widgeons, two Dozen of Larks; let them be all ſing'd and truſs'd up for boiling, blanch them in boiling Water, then throw them out on a Cullender, when cold, lard half of them with ſmall Lard, and either roaſt or fry them brown, as you did your Meat aforeſaid, as quick as you can, becauſe they may not loſe their Goodneſs. When your Meat and Herbs aforeſaid are half-dreſs'd, put your Fowl on the Top of it with the Breaſts down, with as little Broth as barely covers all; then put ſome Broth and Gravy to your fry'd Roots, and ſplit your Hog's Feet aforeſaid, and put into them with a little Bit of Bacon ſtuck with Cloves: Set all a ſtewing together; put likewiſe a Quarter of a Pound of Middling Bacon, ſtuck with two Dozen of Cloves, into the Middle of your Meat that is a ſtewing, and two or three

three Cloves of Garlick, ty'd up in a Rag, a Penyworth of Saffron; you muſt take care in the boiling, that it take not too much Taſte of either: Cover all up, and let it ſtew ſoftly; then make your Thickning ready as followeth: If in Summer, boil up two Quarts of Green Peaſe, and put to them three Pints of good ſtrong Broth, and ſtrain them thro' a Strainer as thick as you can, and thicken your *Olio* with this; but it muſt not be ſo thick as a Cowley for any other Soupe; likewiſe put a little into your fry'd Roots: Or, if in Winter, you may uſe Blue Peaſe; but if you have neither of theſe, put a Quarter of a Pound of Butter in a Sawce-pan, a ſmall Handful of Flower, brown it ſoftly over a clear Fire, rubbing it with a Ladle; when brown, put to it three Pints of the ſame Broth and Gravy, let it boil up, and ſtrain it thro' a fine Sieve; about an Hour before you ſerve it, pour Half of it over your *Olio*, and Half over your fry'd Roots; put into it ſix whole Onions; let all ſtew ſoftly together, giving it a Shake now and then, that it fit not to, and take care that it be tender boil'd, but not coming to a Mash: Set it off before you intend to dish it up, and skim the Fat off clean; then prepare some dry'd Bread in the Bottom of your Dish, a good stout Rim of lean Paste an Inch high, set on with the Yolk of an Egg, and dry'd in an Oven. Then put some of the same Broth from your *Olio* to soak your Bread with. It will take half an Hour's time to dish it in Order; when you dish it up, take up all your Meat, Fowl, and Herbs, in another Dish, and begin with your coarsest Meat first, in the Bottom of your Dish; such as Beef, Pork, mix'd with some of your Roots; lay your first Row out, touching your Rim, and so by degrees draw it into the Top in the Manner of a Sugar-Loaf, the finest of your Fowl next to the Top, with the Hog's Feet and Ears: Then take the fry'd Roots, the Fat being clean taken off, lay them handsomely, with your Spoon, in all the Vacancies and hollow Places round and over your *Olio*; take care you do not hide your Fowl too much

This is Proper for a Wedding supper or Ball.

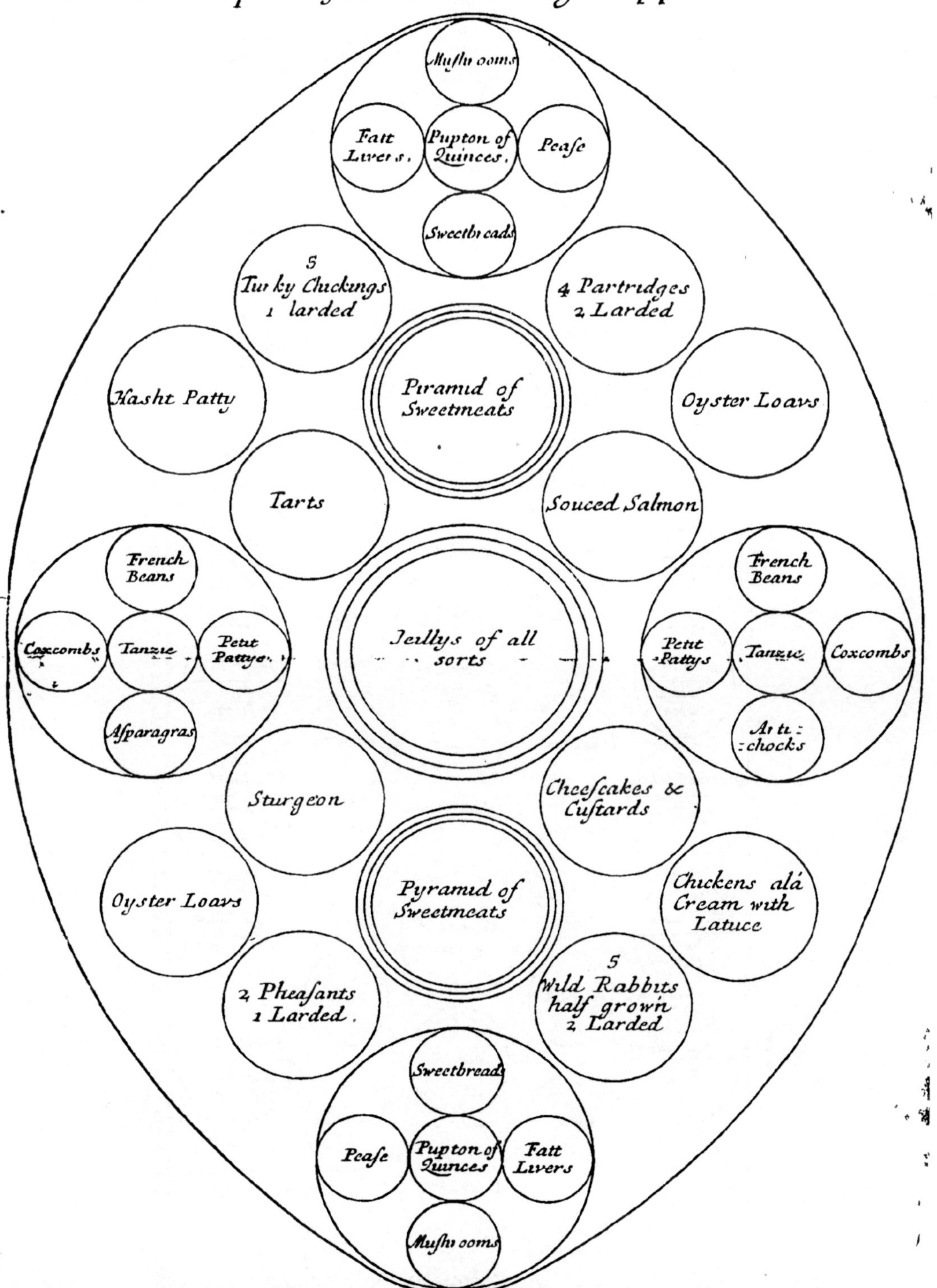

If you please, you may change all the outside Dishes with Sweetmeats or at least you may more the eight small ones, and let the Plates stand, according to the Masters pleasure

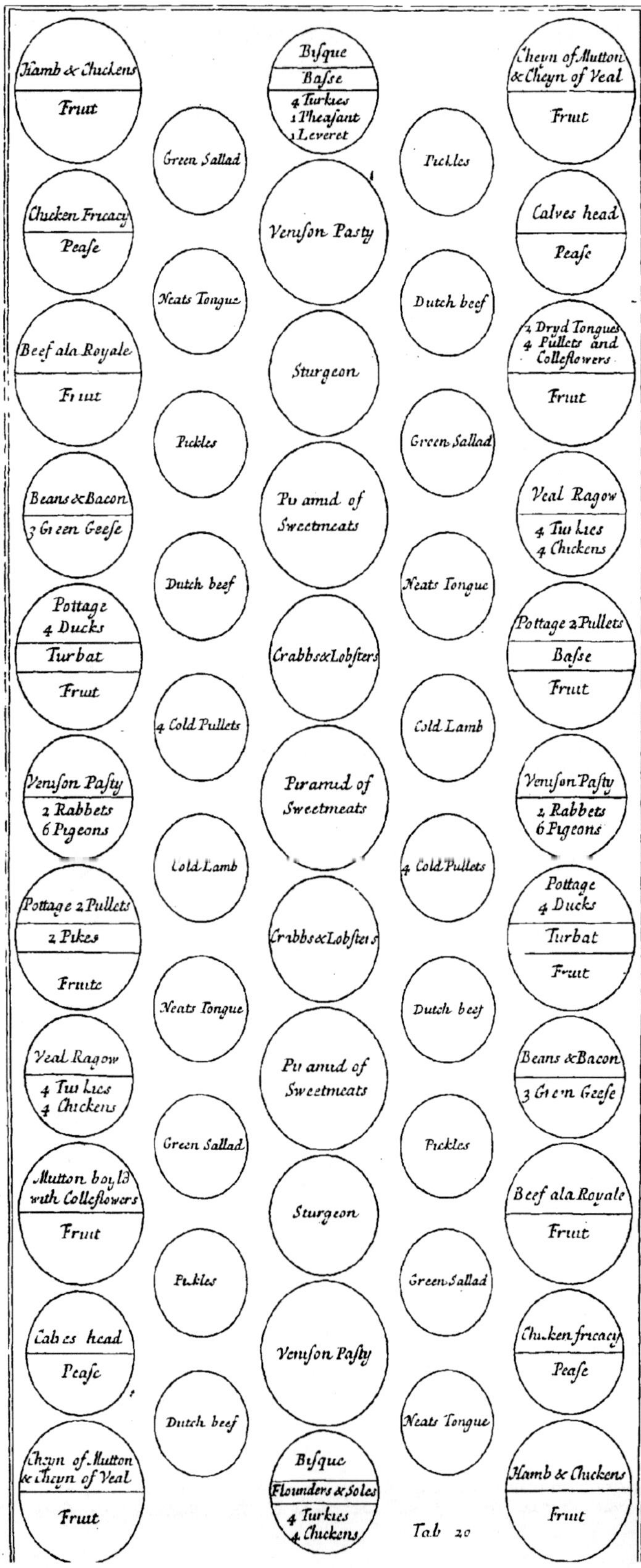

Hamb & Chickens / Fruit	Green Sallad	Biſque / Baſse / 4 Turkies 1 Pheaſant 1 Leveret	Pickles	Cheyn of Mutton & Cheyn of Veal / Fruit
Chicken Fricacy / Peaſe	Neats Tongue	Veniſon Pasty	Dutch beef	Calves head / Peaſe
Beef ala Royale / Fruit	Pickles	Sturgeon	Green Sallad	2 Dryd Tongues 4 Pullets and Colleflowers / Fruit
Beans & Bacon / 3 Green Geeſe	Dutch beef	Piramid of Sweetmeats	Neats Tongue	Veal Ragow / 4 Turkies 4 Chickens
Pottage 4 Ducks / Turbat / Fruit	4 Cold Pullets	Crabbs & Lobſters	Cold Lamb	Pottage 2 Pullets / Baſse / Fruit
Veniſon Paſty / 2 Rabbets 6 Pigeons	Cold Lamb	Piramid of Sweetmeats	4 Cold Pullets	Veniſon Paſty / 2 Rabbets 6 Pigeons
Pottage 2 Pullets / 2 Pikes / Fruite	Neats Tongue	Crabbs & Lobſters	Dutch beef	Pottage 4 Ducks / Turbat / Fruit
Veal Ragow / 4 Turkies 4 Chickens	Green Sallad	Piramid of Sweetmeats	Pickles	Beans & Bacon / 3 Green Geeſe
Mutton boyld with Colleflowers / Fruit	Pickles	Sturgeon	Green Sallad	Beef ala Royale / Fruit
Calves head / Peaſe	Dutch beef	Veniſon Paſty	Neats Tongue	Chicken fricacy / Peaſe
Cheyn of Mutton & Cheyn of Veal / Fruit		Biſque / Flounders & Soles / 4 Turkies 4 Chickens		Hamb & Chickens / Fruit

Tab 20

The three middle Rows of this Table ryſes higher The ſecond Row eight inches higher than the ſides and the Middle eight inches higher than them Rayſed with boards and cover'd handſomly with linnen much, and that you put not too much Broth in your Dish when you dish it up, because you must leave Room for some of your boiling Cowley to be pour'd over it when you serve it away; Then strain the Remainder of your Broth that you stew'd your Roots in, and likewise some of your Stew-pan, be sure there is no Fat on it; put into it the Crust of half a *French* Roll, when it is tender soak'd, put it into a Silver Cup or *China* Bason, with about a Quart of your Broth. So serve it up on a Plate with your *Olio*, as it goes away: Take care you make it not too salt, because there comes Salt from your larded Fowl, and from your Bacon that is stuck with Cloves; take care that none of your Liquor run over the Rim of your Dish; according to your Company and Bigness of your Dish, you may put in half the Quantity above-mention'd. *So serve it.*

To make a Terreyné.

TAKE a ſmall Quantity of all the Ingredients above mention'd in the *Olio*, and ſtew them down after the ſame manner; then place them into your Diſh that you intend to ſerve it in, or in a *Terreyné*-Diſh, if you have one. A *Terreyné*-Diſh, at Court, is made of Silver, round and upright, holding about ſix Quarts *Engliſh* Meaſure, or three Pints and a half *Scotch* Meaſure; with two Handles, ſuch as a ſmall Ciſtern has. If you have a *Terreyné*-Pan, you muſt ſtew it in it an Hour, after you have ſtew'd it down in a Sawce-pan; whereas you put your ſoak'd Bread under your *Olio*, you muſt ſoak it in ſome of the ſame Broth, and put it on the Top of your *Terreyné*, being the Upper Cruſt of —— *French* Rolls; then it will look like the Upper part of a Brown Loaf;

Loaf; but you must be sure to take the Fat off before you put your Bread on, and thicken your Broth a little with Green Pease, strain'd with a little good Broth, the same as you do for Pease Soupe, not quite so thick as a Cream; or you may thicken it with a Cowley. Send it away boiling hot off the Fire; remember to turn up the Breast of your Fowl before you put on your Bread; you may put a larded Sweetbread in the Middle, under your Crust; do not let your *Terreyné*-Pan be fill'd up quite to the Top, because your Cowley ought to swim as high as your Bread. The Butcher-Meat for your *Terreyné* must not be cut in such great Pieces as for your *Olio*, and put in but few Herbs and Roots. You may dish it up after the same Manner, if you have no *Terreyné*-Dish, with a good Rim to hold the Liquor in. Let not your Meat be much higher than your Rim, because it will look too much like an *Olio*, only the Bread being on the Top makes it another thing. To make an Alteration, you may bake it in an Oven, half an Hour before you uſe it, till your Bread and Cowley comes to a Cruſt on the Top of it. We do not uſe to bake it at Court now, but only pour our Cowley hot over the Top of it when you ſerve it; but baking is the good old way, therefore I leave either of them to your Diſcretion. Be ſure clean the Outſide of your *Terreyné*-Diſh. *So ſerve it hot*, Summer or Winter.

To make Forc'd-Meat *that you may uſe in moſt Things of Cookery that require* Forc'd-Meat, *Bottoms of Pies ex cepted, becauſe in theſe, few or no Eggs.*

TAke two Pound of a Leg of Veal, or three, according to your Occaſion, and put to it a Pound of fat Bacon, a Pound

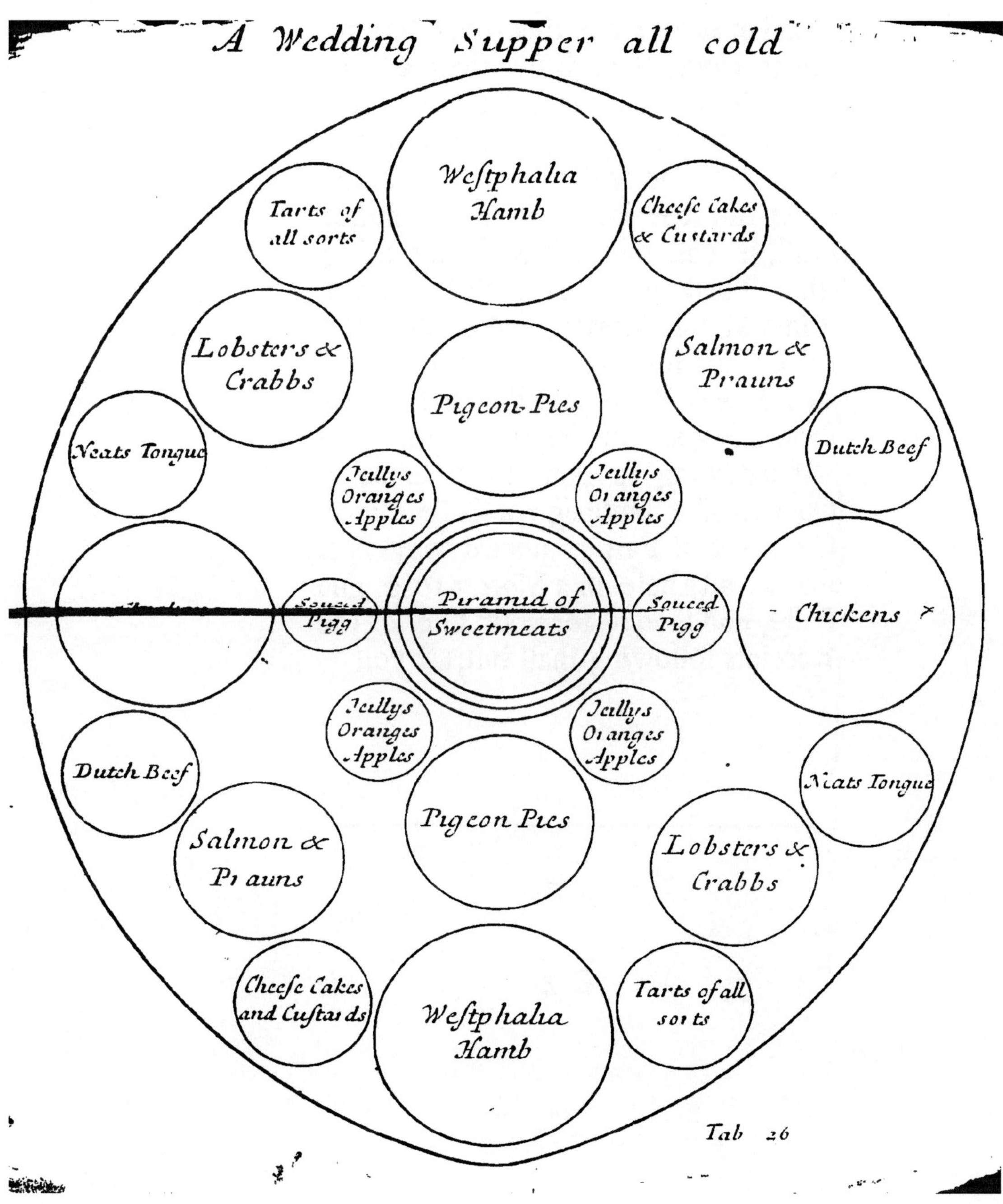
A Wedding Supper all cold
Westphalia Hamb
Tarts of all sorts
Cheese Cakes & Custards
Lobsters & Crabbs
Salmon & Prauns
Pigeon-Pies
Neats Tongue
Dutch Beef
Jellys Oranges Apples
Jellys Oranges Apples
Soused Pigg
Piramid of Sweetmeats
Soused Pigg
Chickens
Jellys Oranges Apples
Jellys Oranges Apples
Dutch Beef
Neats Tongue
Pigeon Pies
Salmon & Prauns
Lobsters & Crabbs
Cheese Cakes and Custards
Westphalia Hamb
Tarts of all sorts
Tab 26

Pound of Sewet; boil them over the Fire half an Hour, then throw them a little in cold Water, that your Fat Bacon run not to Oil in mincing. Then mince them all as fine as Paſte, each by themſelves, for the Bacon will not mince ſmall, if you mince it with any thing elſe. Then mince all together, and put it in a Marble Mortar, and put to it the Ingredients following: The Crum of two *French* Rolls, ſoak'd in Milk or Broth; eight raw Eggs; Pepper and Salt according to your Diſcretion; a Quarter of a Nutmeg; a little minc'd Onion; and Parſley minc'd very fine. Pound all theſe in a Mortar to a fine Paſte, and ſave it for your Uſe, as the Receipts following ſhall inſtruct you.

To make Pullet *or* Chicken-Surprize.

ROast them off; if for a little Diſh, two Chickens, or one Pullet will do. Take the Lean of your Pullet or Chickens from the Bones, and cut it in thin Slices Inch long, and toſs it up in ſix or ſeven Spoonfuls of Milk or Cream, with the Bigneſs of half an Egg of Butter; ſcrape a Nutmeg, Pepper and Salt, thicken it with a little Duſt of Flower, to the Thickneſs of a good Cream, then boil it up and ſet it to cool; then cut ſix or ſeven thin Slices of Bacon, and round; Place them in a Patty-pan, and put on each Slice ſome of the Forc'd Meat aforeſaid, and work them up in Form of a *French* Roll, with a raw Egg in your Hand, leaving them a little Hollow in the Middle; then

then put in your Fowl, and cover them on the Top with ſome of the ſame Forc'd Meat, rubbing it ſmooth over with your Hand, and an Egg; make them of the Height and Bigneſs of a *French* Roll; throw a little fine grated Bread over; bake them three Quarters of an Hour in a gentle Oven, or under a Baking-Cover, bake them to a yellow Brown; place them on your Mazarine, that they may not touch one another, ſo that they may not fall flat in the baking: But you may form them on your Kitchen-Table with your Slices of Bacon under them; then lift them up with your broad Kitchen-Knife, and place them on that which you intend to bake them on. Let your Sawce be Butter and Gravy, and ſqueez'd Lemon, and your Garniſhing fry'd Parſley, and cut Orange; you may put the Legs of one of your Chickens into the Sides of one of your Loaves that you intend to put in the Middle of your Diſh. This is proper for a Side-Diſh, for Firſt Courſe in Summer or Winter, where you can have the Ingredients above-mention'd.

To make Rabbet-Surprize.

ROAST off two or three half grown Rabbets, according to the Bignefs of your Difh; cut off the Heads, clofe by the Shoulder, and the firft Joint of the Hind-Legs; then cut all the lean Meat from the Back-Bones, and cut it, and tofs it up as you did for your Pullet-Surprize; then take the Quantity of Forc'd Meat aforefaid, and tofs it up likewife, and place all round each of the Rabbets aforefaid, leaving a long Trough in the Back open, that you think will hold the Meat you cut out, with the Sawce; then cover it with the fame Forc'd Meat, fmooth'd as well as you can with your Hand and a raw Egg, fquare at both Ends, throw a little grated Bread; then butter a Mazarine or Patty-pan, and take them from your Dreffer, where you form'd them, and

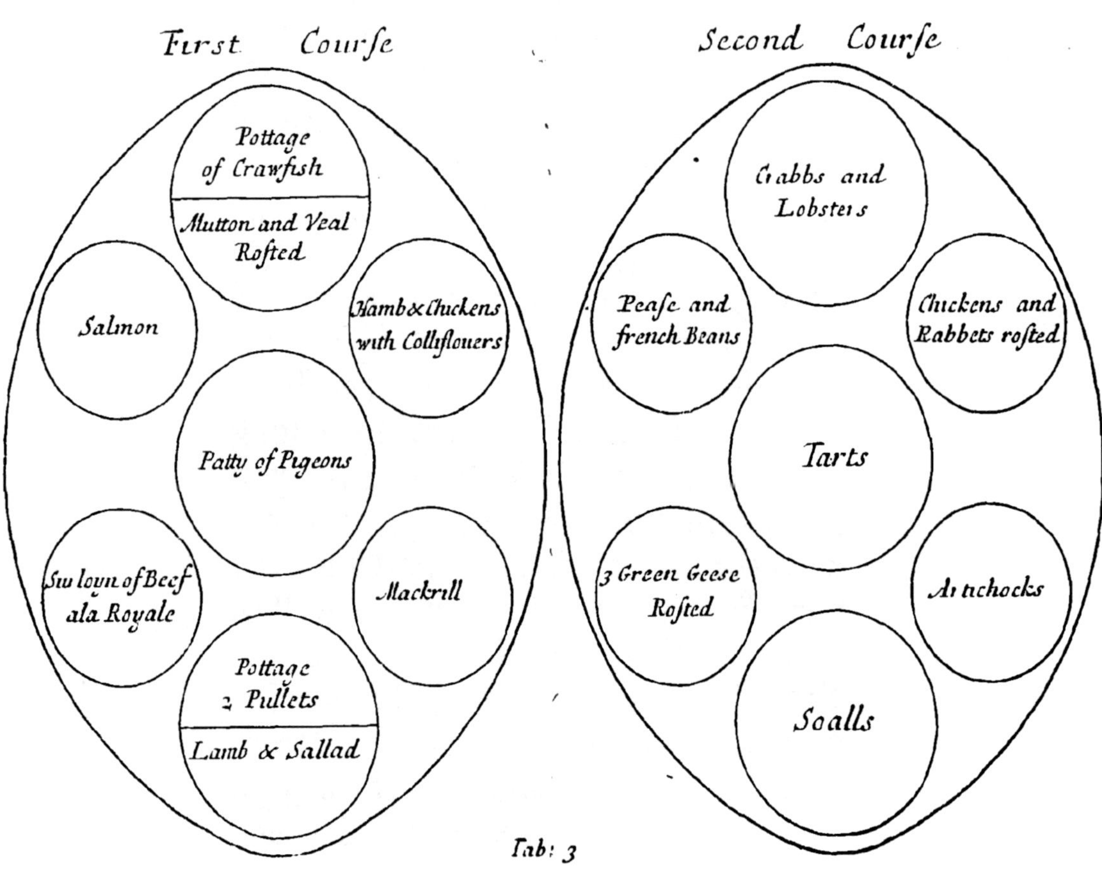

First Course
Pottage of Crawfish
Mutton and Veal Rosted
Salmon
Hamb & Chickens with Colliflouers
Patty of Pigeons
Sirloyn of Beef ala Royale
Mackrill
Pottage 2 Pullets
Lamb & Sallad
Second Course
Crabbs and Lobsters
Pease and french Beans
Chickens and Rabbets rosted
Tarts
3 Green Geese Rosted
Artichocks
Soalls
Tab: 3

and place thereon: Bake them three Quarters of an Hour before you ſerve them; when they are of a gentle Brown. Let your Sawce be Butter, Gravy and Lemon; and your Garniſhing Orange, and fry'd Parſley. *So ſerve it* for firſt Courſe.

To make Pupton *of* Pigeons.

FOR a little Diſh, you may take ſix Pigeons if not more, according to the Bigneſs of your Diſh, truſs them, ſwing and blanch them; then fry them off in a little Butter, or Hog's Lard, being firſt larded with ſmall Lard; then put them a ſtewing with a little Broth or Gravy; when they are almoſt tender, put to them two Sweetbreads cut in large Bits and fry'd, a Handful of Morils, and Muſhrooms well pick'd and waſh'd, twelve Cheſnuts blanch'd: Put all together, then take a Sawce-pan with

with a Quarter of a Pound of Butter, a ſmall Handful of Flower, two whole Onions; brown it over the Fire with a Pint of Gravy, put in your Ingredients aforeſaid, being well ſeaſon'd with Pepper, Salt and Nutmeg. Let it ſtew till moſt of your Ragoo ſticks to your Meat, then ſet it off of the Fire a cooling. Take a Patty-pan or Sawce-pan, and butter the Bottom and Sides; then cut four or five Slices of Bacon as long as your Hand, as thin as a Shilling, and place them at the Bottom and Sides of your Pan at an equal Diſtance; then place all over it a Quantity of the ſame Forc'd Meat aforeſaid, half Inch thick, as high on the Sides of your Pan as you think will hold your Pigeons and Ragoo. Then pour in your cold Ragoo and Pigeons, placing them with the Breaſts to the Bottom of the Pan, becauſe the Bottom Side is turn'd up when it goes to the Table; then take out your whole Onion, Bacon, and Cloves that was in your Brown, and ſqueeze in a whole Lemon, place your Pigeons with the Breaſts to the Middle of the

Pan,

Pan, and your Ragoo plac'd betwixt your Pigeons at an equal Diſtance. Then cover it all over with the ſame Forc'd Meat Inch thick, and cloſe it well round the Sides, ſmooth it well with your Hand and an Egg; ſtrew a little grated Bread, then bake it an Hour before you have Occaſion; then looſe it from your Patty-pan or Sawce-pan from the Sides with your Knife, then put it on your Mazarine or little Diſh, wherein you intend to ſerve it, and turn it Upſide down clearly; if it is well bak'd, it will ſtand upright like a brown Loaf. Squeeze over it an Orange, lay round it fry'd Parſley; the Sawce is in the Middle. *So ſerve it* for firſt Courſe. You may make Pupton of Larks the ſame way, only adding the Yolks of hard-boil'd Eggs.

To make Veal *or* Mutton-Cutlets, à la Maintenon.

CUT your Cutlets handſome, and beat them thin with your Cleaver, and ſeaſon them with a little Pepper and Salt; then lay all over them ſome of the aforeſaid Forc'd Meat, except two Inches of the Rib-bone, and ſmooth it over with your Knife, to the Thickneſs of a Crown; then take as many half Sheets of Writing Paper as you have Cutlets, and butter them with melted Butter on one Side; likewiſe dip your Stake in melted Butter, and throw a little grated Bread on the Top of your Forc'd Meat all round, a Stake on each Half Sheet of Paper croſs the Middle of it, leaving the Bone about an Inch out; then cloſe the Two Ends of your Paper, cloſing it on the Sides

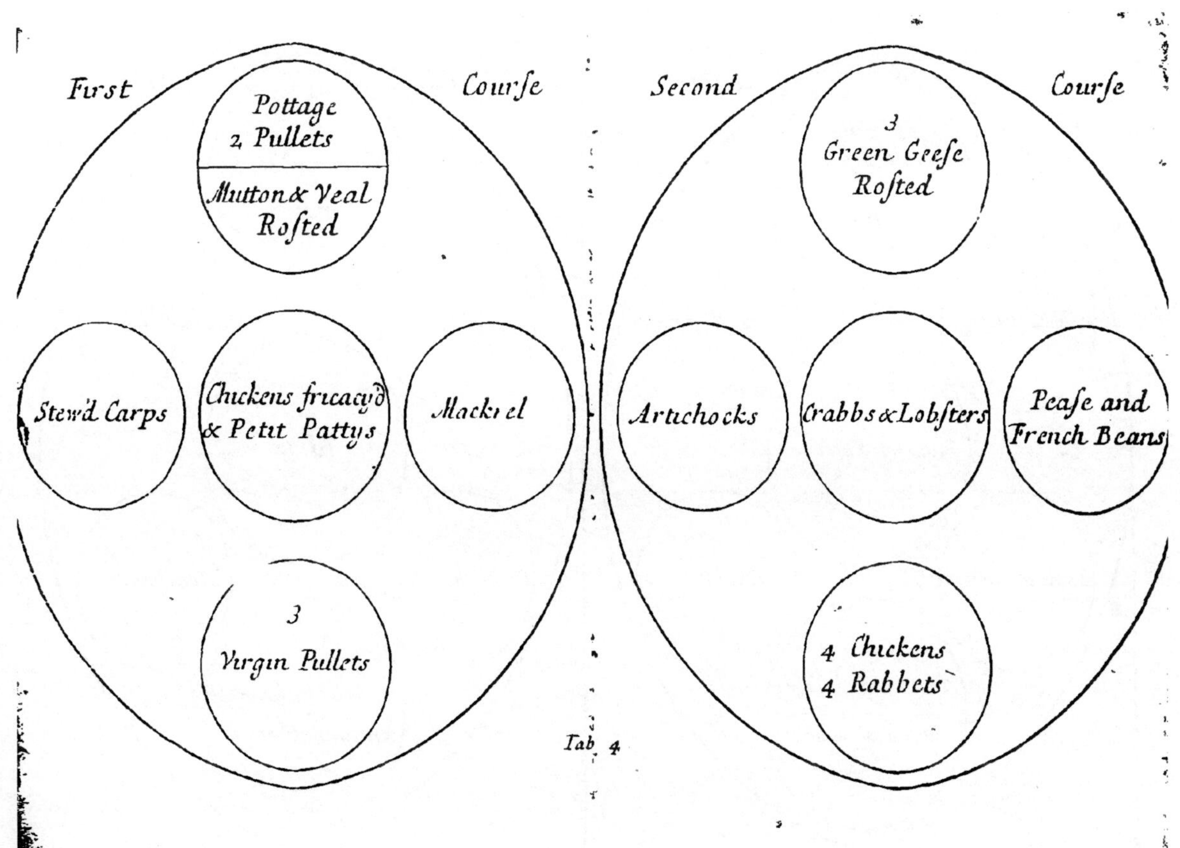
First
Course
Pottage
2 Pullets
Mutton & Veal
Rosted
Stew'd Carps
Chickens fricacy'd
& Petit Pattys
Mackrel
3
Virgin Pullets
Second
Course
3
Green Geese
Rosted
Artichocks
Crabbs & Lobsters
Pease and
French Beans
4 Chickens
4 Rabbets
Tab 4

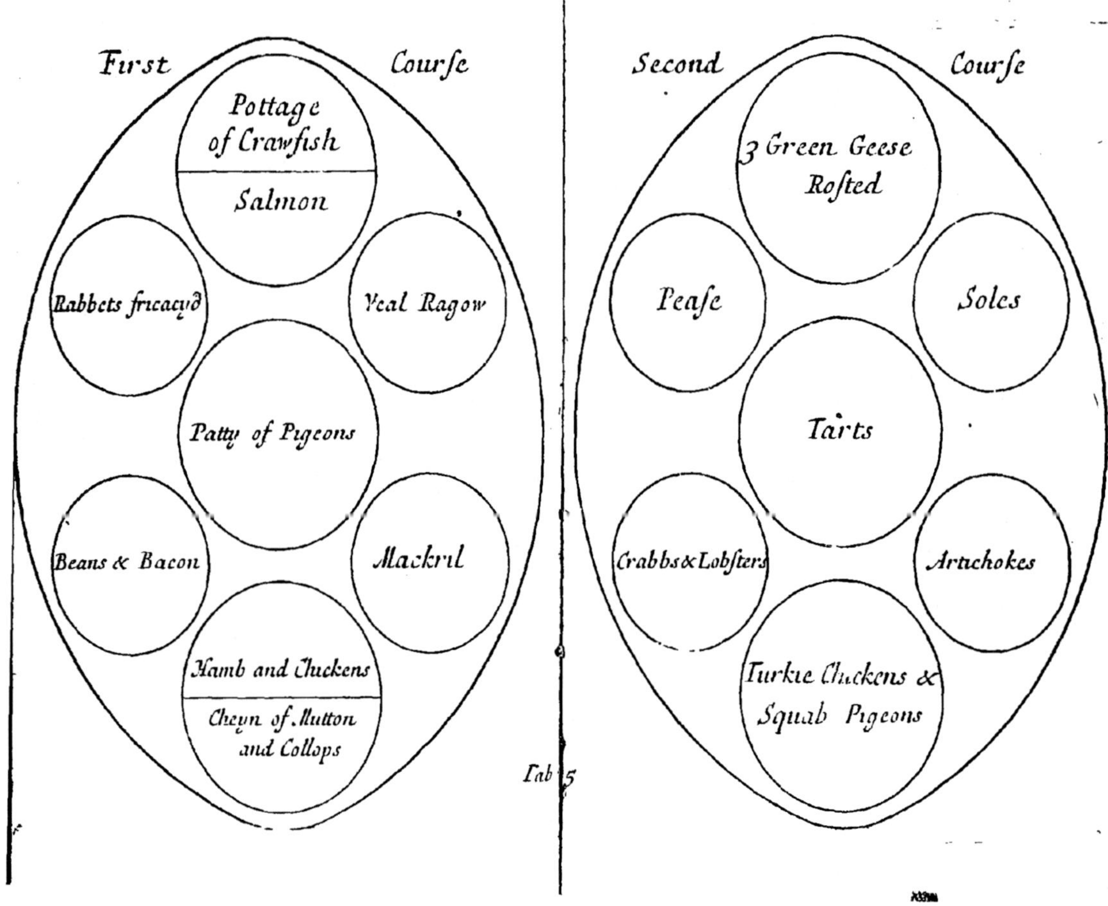
First Course
Pottage of Crawfish
Salmon
Rabbets fricacy'd
Veal Ragow
Patty of Pigeons
Beans & Bacon
Mackril
Hamb and Chickens
Cheyn of Mutton and Collops
Tab 5
Second Course
3 Green Geese Rosted
Pease
Soles
Tarts
Crabbs & Lobsters
Artichokes
Turkie Chickens & Squab Pigeons

as you do a Turn-over Tart. Cut off your waſte Paper; So broil them half an Hour before you ſerve them: But of Veal three Quarters. You may take the Paper, half of them for one Side of your Diſh, lay them round with the Bones out. Let your Sawce be Butter, Gravy and Lemon.

To Ragoo Turkey *or* Gooſe.

SWing them and beat them down with a Cleaver, flat them, blanch them off in boiling Water, and, when cold, lard them thro' with good big Lard, as big as two Quills; but firſt ſeaſon your Lard with Pepper, Salt, Nutmeg, and beaten Cloves; then ſeaſon your Turkey or Gooſe, Outſide and Inſide, as you do for a Pie, and place in the Bottom

tom of your Braſs Diſh or great Sawce-pan, a Pound of Sewet cut in Slices, and half a Pound of Bacon cut in Slices: Then flower the Breaſts of your Fowl, turn it down in your Sawce-pan; ſet it a ſtewing two Hours, before you want it, over a clear Fire; put into it, at firſt, half a Pint of your fat Broth or Gravy, then let it ſtew ſoftly till it comes to a good Colour; put to it two whole Onions, two Bay-Leaves, and a Sprig of Thyme: Cover it with a Baking Cover, with a little clear Fire over the Top; you muſt look on it frequently that it burn not. When the Breaſt is of a Brownneſs to your Mind, then turn the Back down, adding to it a little Broth or Gravy, till it is ſtew'd tender. At the ſame time, put over the Fire, with another Sawce-pan, a Quarter of a Pound of Butter, a little Handful of Flower, two Onions; rub it ſoftly till it comes to a good Brown, then put to it a Quart of good Gravy. If in Winter time, your Ragoo may be Carrots, Turneps and Onions, cut the Bigneſs of the Yolk of an Egg, fry'd in in Hog's Lard, or clarify'd Butter. But first half-boil them, to take away the Over-ſtrongneſs of your Roots and Onions, and boil them tender in your aforeſaid Sawce; then put it over your Gooſe or Turkey, firſt taking the Fat off, and ſqueezing in half a Lemon; boil it up to a moderate thickneſs, little thicker than a Cream: If your Fowls are of a good Colour, put your Ragoo under them, none over. Let your Garniſhing be fry'd Bread, cut in ſmall Bits, and fry'd Parſley betwixt. You may ragoo any Fowl after the ſame manner, or Butchers Meat. This Ragoo is proper for a Rump of Beef, or a Surloin, Ox-head, or a Gigget of Mutton, or Breaſt of Veal. But this Ragoo is not proper for ſmall Fowl, if you are in a Country where you can have any thing elſe. But for a Change, take for ſmall Fowl, Morils, green or dry'd Muſhrooms, according to the Seaſon of the Year, Aſparagus cut Inch long, or Cheſnuts. All, or any of theſe, may ſerve at a time, as the Country can afford, or you may uſe a few Forc'd-Meat

Balls, ſtew'd off in your Sawce. Let your Garniſhing be according to your Fancy. *So ſerve it* for firſt Courſe.

To make a Leer *of* Fiſh Sawce, *after the* Engliſh *Way.*

FOR a Cod's Head blanch off a Quart of Oyſters, then ſave your Liquor, waſh your Oyſters in Water, cleaning them from the Beards and Shells. But in place of Oyſters, take two or three Lobſters, and cut them in large Dices; place either of them in a Sawce-pan: If your Cod's Head is large, you muſt put two Pound of Butter to it, if ſmall, one Pound. You muſt put to each Pound of Butter, the Yolks of three Eggs, three Anchovies taken from the Bones, and minc'd ſmall, one Lemon, ſcrape a Nutmeg, a little beaten Pepper, and whole Onion, a Bunch of ſweet

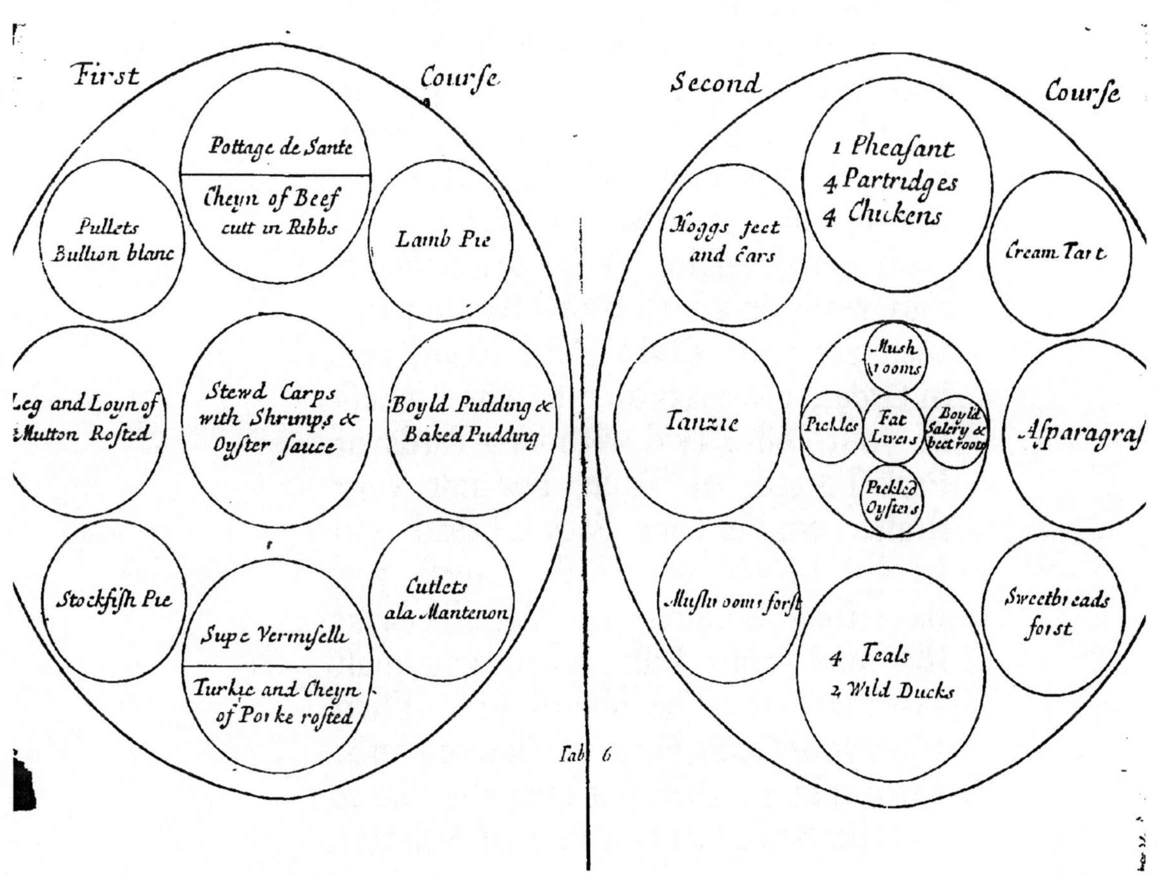

First Course
Pottage de Sante
Cheyn of Beef cutt in Ribbs
Pullets Bullion blanc
Lamb Pie
Leg and Loyn of Mutton Rosted
Stewd Carps with Shrimps & Oyster sauce
Boyld Pudding & Baked Pudding
Stockfish Pie
Cutlets ala Mantenon
Supe Vermiselli
Turkie and Cheyn of Porke rosted
Second Course
1 Pheasant
4 Partridges
4 Chickens
Hoggs feet and Ears
Cream Tart
Tanzie
Mush rooms
Pickles
Fat Livers
Boyld Salery & beet roots
Pickled Oysters
Asparagras
Mushrooms forst
4 Teals
2 Wild Ducks
Sweetbreads forst

Tab 6

ſweet Herbs, ty'd up together with Pack Thread. Let your ſweet Herbs be a Sprig of Thyme, half a Bay-Leaf, and a little Parſley: If you have Oyſters, put your aforeſaid Liquor to them that came from your Oyſters when they were ſet off; but if you have Lobſters, take the Spawn, or Red out of the Body; or if they have neither Spawn nor Red, take the ſmall Claws, and pound them in a Mortar, and ſtrain it out with five or ſix Spoonfuls of *White-Wine* or Gravy, and put to your Butter and Ingredients aforeſaid. Your Sawce being thus ready in a well tinn'd Sawce-pan; then get your Cod's Head clean, and in Order, cut according to the Bigneſs of your Diſh; ty'd with two Yards of Pack-Thread, or Tape, but not very ſtrait, becauſe your Pack-Thread will be apt to cut your Fiſh, unleſs you have ſome Splinters of Wood betwixt that and your Fiſh, when you muſt take care they be not of Fir. Then place your Cod's Head in a Sawce-pan or earthen Pan; then put over the Fire in another Sawce-pan, a Pint of Vinegar, and a Spoonful of whole Pepper and Cloves, a green Lemon Peel, two Bay-Leaves, three or four Onions in Slices, two Handfuls of Salt. Let all this boil up together, and pour it over your Cod's Head. Let it lie in Pickle an Hour before you boil it, turning it frequently, that it may take the Taſte of the Pickle; then having a Pan of Water over the Fire to boil it in, if your Cod's Head is tolerably big, it will take an Hour's ſoft boiling. Put it in with a Fiſh-Plate under it, if you have one; if not, you may put a Mazarine under it, and boil the Pickle with it, adding a Handful or two of Salt, as you find Occaſion, according to your Diſcretion. Take care you take it up with a good ſtrong Skimmer under your Mazarine, without Breaking. Put it a draining on a Cullender. At the ſame time, draw up your Sawce aforeſaid over a gentle clear Fire, ſtirring it with a wooden or well-turn'd Ladle, as you do to draw up Butter: Let it be thicker than a Cream. If you find it is too thin, ſhake a little Flower on your Ladle, and if it

is

is too thick, add a Spoonful or two of *White Wine* or Gravy; then take out the Bundle of ſweet Herbs, and whole Onions, and ſqueeze your Lemon; then place ſome Sippets about your Diſh, and ſome in the Bottom; then ſlide in your Cod's Head, being well drain'd, with his Back up; You may pour a little of your Fiſh Sawce on your Cod's Head while it is a draining, to make the Water go from it. Let your Garniſhing be ſcrap'd *Horſe-Radiſh*, and pickled Barberries or Lemon; your Sawce being very hot, pour it over. *So ſerve it.* But if you have Plenty of Fiſh, you may garniſh it with fry'd Smelts, or Sparlings turn'd round, or you may uſe Whitings fry'd, and Parſley betwixt them. Dip your Fiſh that is to fry into two raw Eggs, and then with fine grated Bread, and a little Salt, and fry them in Clarify'd Butter or Hog's Lard. *So ſerve it.* I have been the more particular in this Receipt, becauſe you may do any other ſtrong Fiſh after the ſame Manner. As for Example, *Salmon*, *Pike*, *Trout*, or whatever you have. If *Sal-*

mon or *Trout*, uſe no Vinegar, becauſe it takes the Colour away.

To do Pike-Cabilow *after the* Dutch *Way*.

SCale it and take the Guts out; being clean waſh'd, cut off its Head. But it is convenient this Pike be pretty large, and cut in Slices with a ſharp Knife, about a little Inch thick; if you can cut the Joint of the Back,it will be much eaſier cut: When you come within a Span of the Tail,cut it thro' the Bone, and leave the Fiſh whole on the Underſide, that it may hang together: Then throw it all into a Pan of cold Water. If your Fiſh is new, it will crimp,and eat as hard as the Kernel of a Nut. It is admir'd by thoſe that have travel'd in the Country. Boil it in good Store of Water, and ſalt it pretty high;

high; when it boils up, pour in a Quarter of a Pint of Vinegar, skim it very clean, ſplit your Head in two; put it a boiling with your Tail, five or ſix Minutes; before you put in your Slices and Milt, take the Gall out of it; boil your Slices well for a Quarter of an Hour: Being drain'd, place the Head and Tail in the Middle of your Diſh, laying the Slices round with ſome Sippets under. In *Holland*, the Sawce is only oil'd Butter, melted gently over the Fire, and ſtirr'd about with a Ladle, and ſo pour'd over, for their Butter is as thick oil'd, as ours is drawn up. But for the Queen, we draw our Butter up. A Pound of Butter, with a Spoonful of Water, drawn up, is as thick as a Cream, ſqueeze a Lemon, *and ſo ſerve it hot.* Let your Garniſhing be a little Parſley pick'd fine and waſh'd, and laid round. We likewiſe do Salmon ſo, but it will take more Boiling, but no Vinegar in the Boiling. And, likewiſe, we do freſh Cod ſo, when they are very new. When you have freſh Cod, boil the Livor with it, and take care you do not over-boil your Slices; for it will boil as ſoon as your Pike, or rather ſooner: But the Head and Livor will take half an Hour, and the Tail little leſs. But for this, they take only half-grown Cods. Then let your Sawce be as aforeſaid. *So ſerve it.*

To do a Haddock *the* Dutch *Way.*

BEING ſcal'd and gutted, and very freſh, ſcore them with a ſharp Knife into the Back-Bone on both ſides, and throw them into cold Water an Hour before you boil them in Salt, and Water, and Vinegar. They will boil in leſs than half an Hour, but that according to the Bigneſs, only to that degree that they will come from the Bone, this you muſt do according to Judgment. Then for your Sawce, take Turneps,

Turneps, and cut them as ſmall as Yolks of Eggs, and boil them tender in Water and Salt. In *Holland* they boil 'em with the Fiſh, and they take very little more Boiling than the Fiſh, becauſe they are better than ours; but if you boil *Engliſh* Turneps, you muſt boil 'em a little before you put in your Fiſh; but you muſt not boil your Turneps ſo tender, as if they were to eat with Beef or Mutton; then drain them from the Liquor, and put two or three Dozen of Turneps, according to the Bigneſs of your Diſh, into a Pound of drawn Butter, and a little fine minc'd Parſley: So put your Haddocks in your Diſh, and Sippets under them, and pour your Turneps and Sawce over; and throw a little minc'd Parſley about your Diſh. *So ſerve it.* You may do Whitings or Shoals the ſame way.

To

To do Scate *or* Thornback, *the* Dutch *or* Englifh *Way.*

SKin them on both Sides, then cut the two Sides from the Body, and cut each Side down thro' the Middle with your Knife; then lay each half crofs-ways, and cut it in Slices crofs-ways, half Inch thick. When you come up toward the thick Part, cut it thinner; Throw it in cold Water with the Livor, an Hour or two before you boil it. If your Fifh is frefh, it will make it curdle and turn crimp. Then boil it in a Brafs-Difh, with Water, Salt, and Vinegar; skim it well in the Boiling; Put your Livor a boiling two or three Minutes before you put in your cut Fifh: Half a Quarter of an Hour will boil your cut Fifh; Take up your Slices carefully, that you break

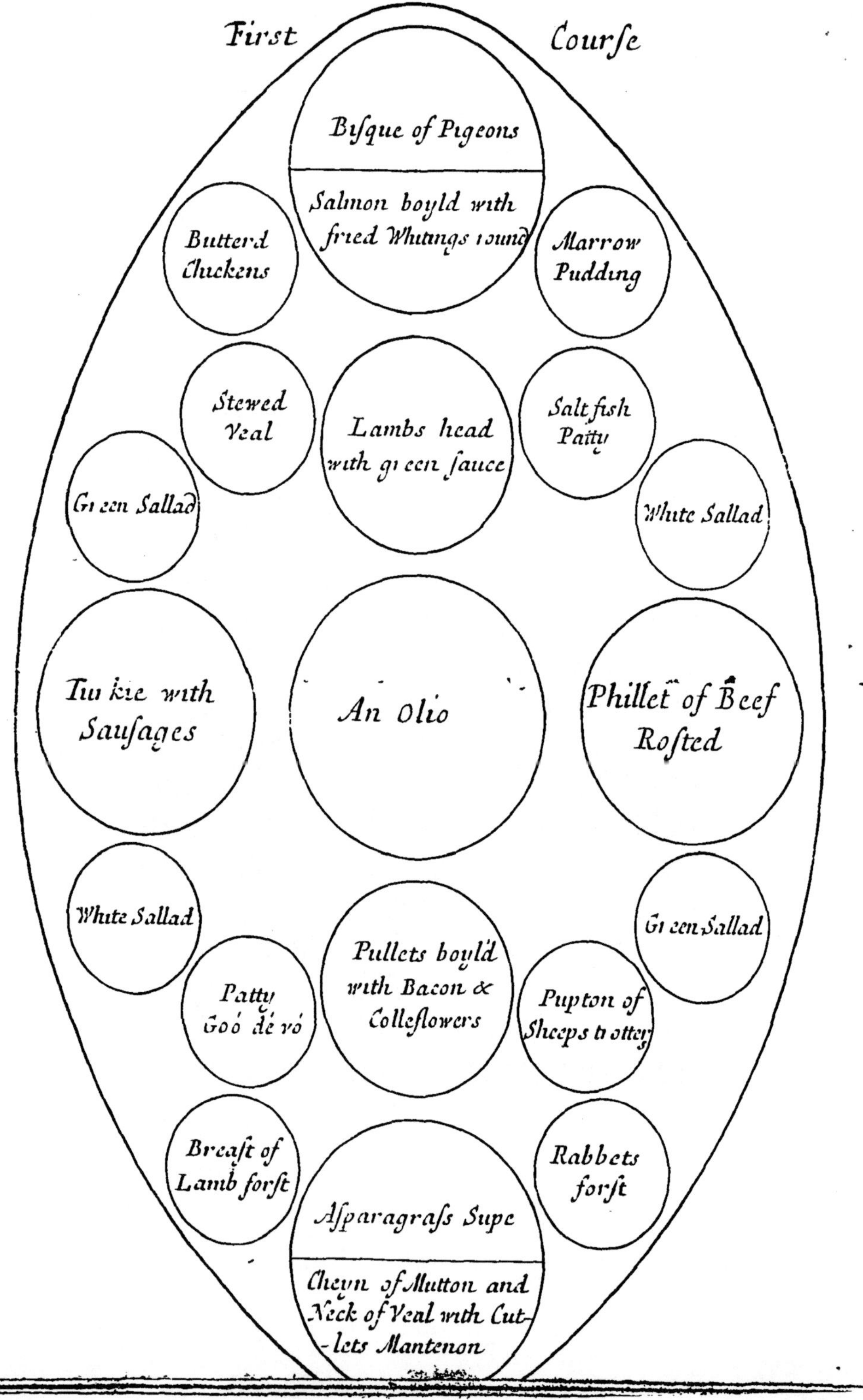
First Course
Bisque of Pigeons
Salmon boyld with fried Whitings round
Butterd Chickens
Marrow Pudding
Stewed Veal
Lambs head with green sauce
Saltfish Patty
Green Sallad
White Sallad
Turkie with Sausages
An Olio
Phillet of Beef Rosted
White Sallad
Green Sallad
Pullets boyl'd with Bacon & Colleflowers
Patty Goó dé vó
Pupton of Sheeps trotters
Breast of Lamb forst
Rabbets forst
Asparagrass Supe
Cheyn of Mutton and Neck of Veal with Cut-lets Mantenon

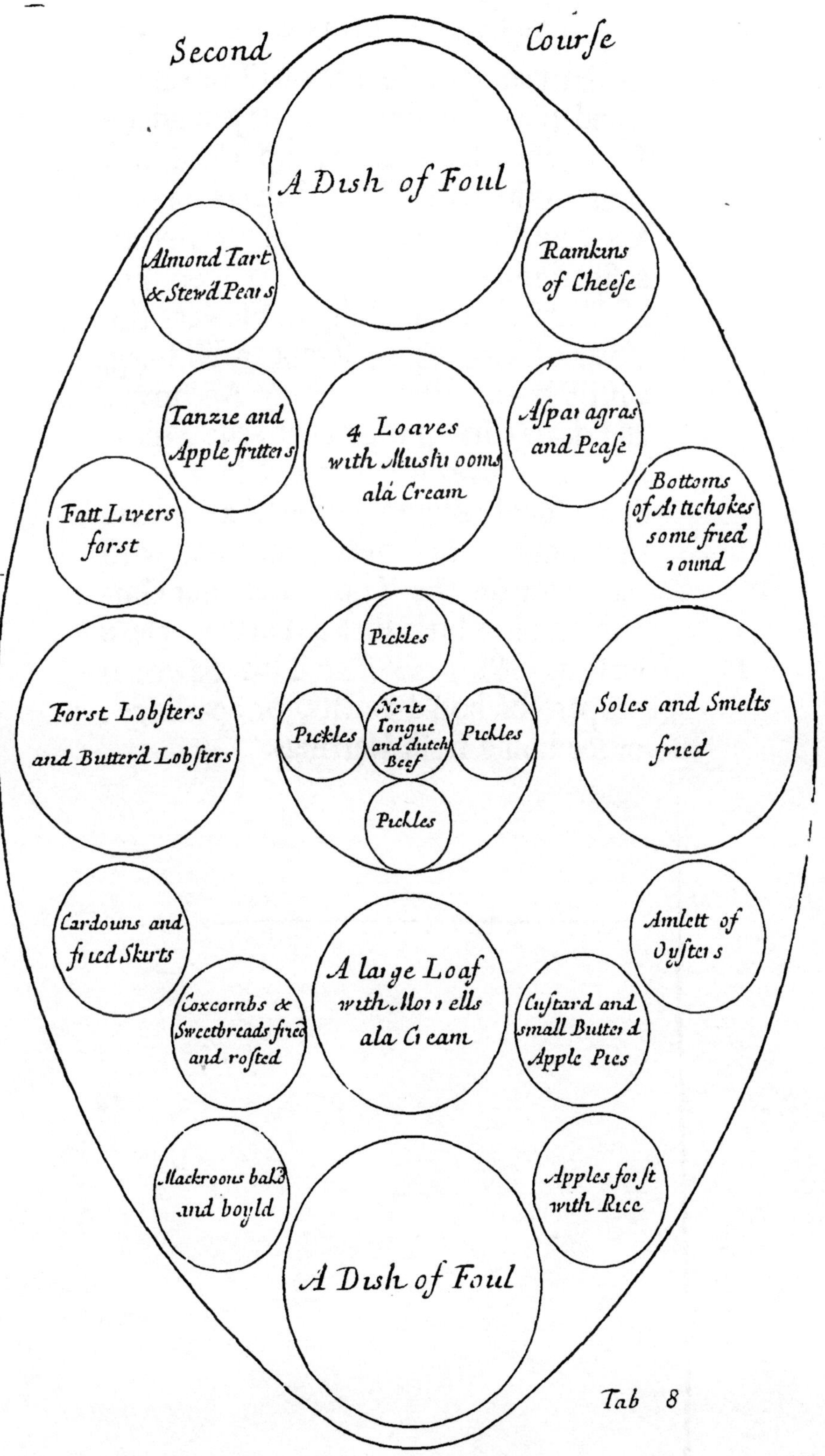
Second Course
A Dish of Foul
Almond Tart & Stew'd Pears
Ramkins of Cheese
Tanzie and Apple fritters
4 Loaves with Mushrooms ala Cream
Aspar agras and Pease
Fatt Livers forst
Bottoms of Artichokes some fried round
Pickles
Forst Lobsters and Butter'd Lobsters
Pickles
Neats Tongue and dutch Beef
Pickles
Soles and Smelts fried
Pickles
Cardouns and fried Skirts
Amlett of Oysters
A large Loaf with Morrells ala Cream
Coxcombs & Sweetbreads fried and rosted
Custard and small Butter'd Apple Pies
Mackroons bak'd and boyld
Apples forst with Rice
A Dish of Foul
Tab 8

break them not; for they will be turn'd round like a Hoop, and very tender; Then when it's drain'd, ſlip them into your Diſh, with ſome Sippets under. Let your Sawce be a Pound of Butter, a Spoonful of Vinegar, two Spoonfuls of Water, a little Duſt of Flawer, the Yolks of two Eggs, ſcrape a Nutmeg, a little beaten Pepper, minc'd Anchovy; and draw this up together to the Thickneſs of a Cream; then put in a good Spoonful of Muſtard, and half a Lemon; then pour it hot over your Fiſh, with the Livor on the Top. Let your Garniſhing be a little Pick'd Parſley, clean waſh'd. *So ſerve it.* This Sawce is proper for boil'd Smelts, or Sparlings; or for boil'd freſh Herrings.

To make Spinnage-Roſolis.

TAKE for a Plate the Bigneſs of two Eggs of boil'd Spinnage, ſqueeze it well from the Water, mince it fine, and put to it the Bigneſs of a Yolk of an Egg of Sugar, as big as half a Yolk of Butter, two Spoonfuls of Cream, mince an Ounce of Cordicitron very ſmall, the Yolks of two hard Eggs, a little Salt, ſcrape a Nutmeg, a little beaten Cinnamon; warm all theſe Ingredients over the Fire in a Sawce-pan; Set it to cool, and make a Paſte as followeth. Take two raw Eggs, two Spoonfuls of Milk, a little Salt, the Bigneſs of a Nutmeg of Sugar, work this to a Paſte of Flower, and roll it up as thin as for a Tart, rather thinner Cut your Paſte in ſquare Pieces, as big as the Palm of your Hand, and lay on each Piece a

Spoonful

Spoonful of your aforesaid Ingredients, wetting your Paste round the Spinnage. Turn half the Paste over the Spinnage, and pinch it handsomely round, Half-Moon Fashion, close it well with your Finger, that it open not in Dressing; cut it round with a Runner or Jagg. You may fry them in Hog's Lard or Clarify'd Butter, as you do Fritters; or you may boil them in boiling Water; a Quarter of an Hour will boil them. If they are boil'd, when you dish them up, you may throw over them a little grated Bread and Cheese; if they are fry'd, grate only a little Sugar over them. They are proper for second Course in a little Dish or Plate; or for Supper. *So serve it.*

To make Marrow-Puddings *in Skins, the* Engliſh *Way.*

TAke the Crum of four *French* Rolls, half a Pound of coarſe Bisket; Cut your *French* Rolls in Slices, put them in an earthen Pan or Sawce-pan; put over the Fire two Quarts of Milk till it's blood-warm, and pour it over your Bread; cover it cloſe up till it is cold, then take a Pound of Marrow, rub your Bread and Milk aforeſaid thro' a Cullender with a wooden Ladle. Your Marrow being minc'd, put them together with five Eggs beaten up very fine, and ſtrain'd thro' a Strainer or Cloth, to keep out the Tread, and put to your Bread aforeſaid. Seaſon with a little Sugar, according to your Diſcretion, as you do another Pudding, ſcrape in

half

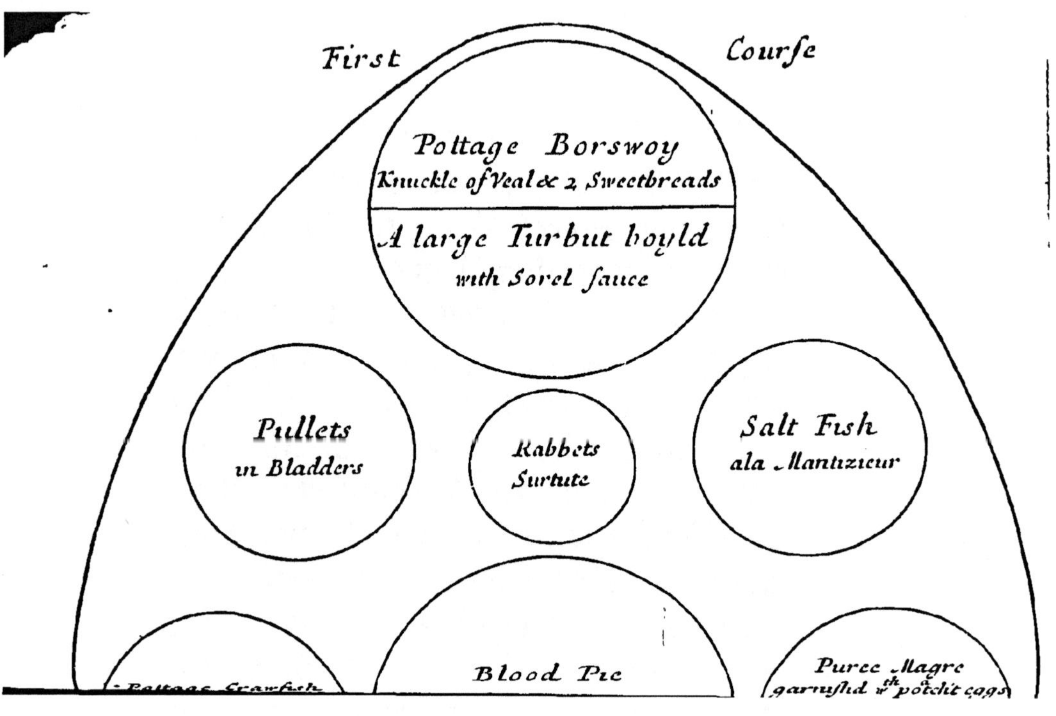
First Course
Pottage Borswoy
Knuckle of Veal & 2 Sweetbreads
A large Turbut boyld
with Sorel sauce
Pullets
in Bladders
Rabbets
Surtute
Salt Fish
ala Mantizieur
Blood Pie
Puree Magre
garnishd wth potcht eggs

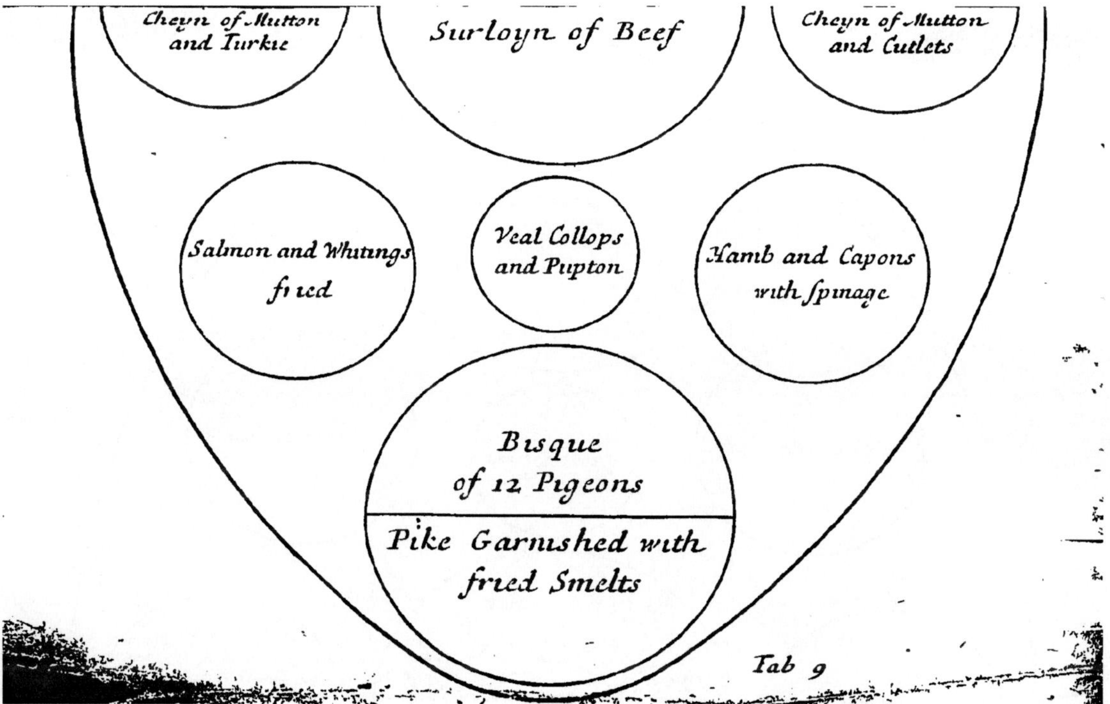
Cheyn of Mutton
and Turkie
Surloyn of Beef
Cheyn of Mutton
and Cutlets
Salmon and Whitings
fried
Veal Collops
and Pupton
Hamb and Capons
with ſpinage
Bisque
of 12 Pigeons
Pike Garnished with
fried Smelts
Tab 9

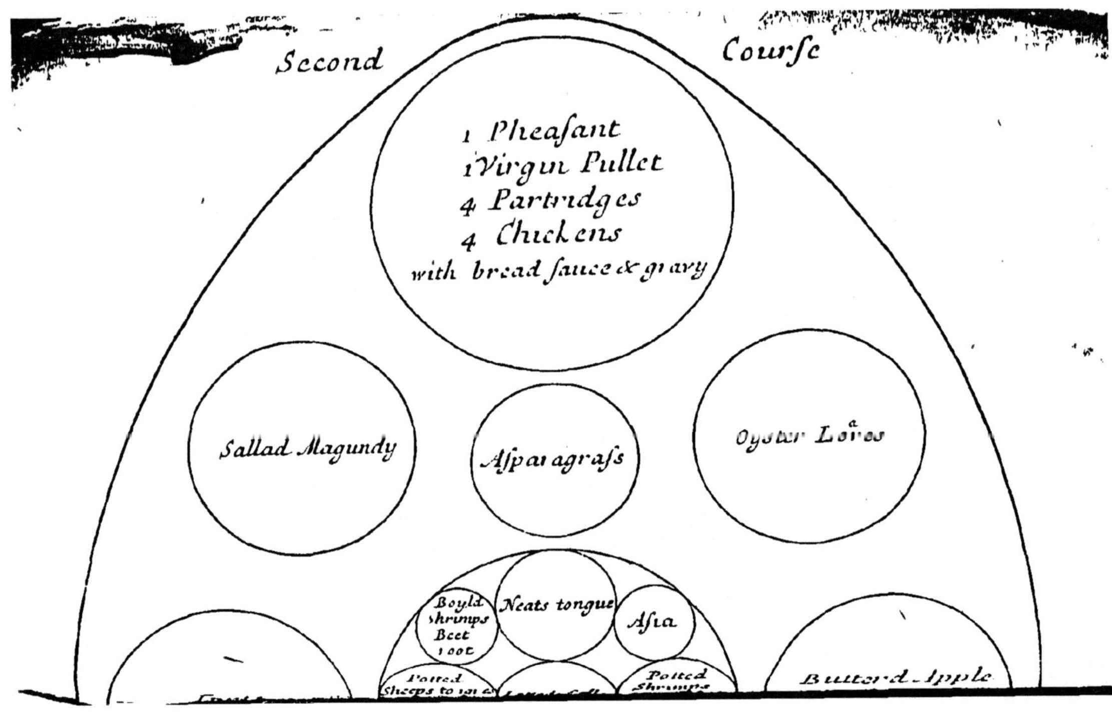
Second Course
1 Pheasant
1 Virgin Pullet
4 Partridges
4 Chickens
with bread sauce & gravy
Sallad Magundy
Asparagrass
Oyster Loaves
Boyld shrimps
Beet root
Neats tongue
Asia
Potted
Potted
Butterd Apple

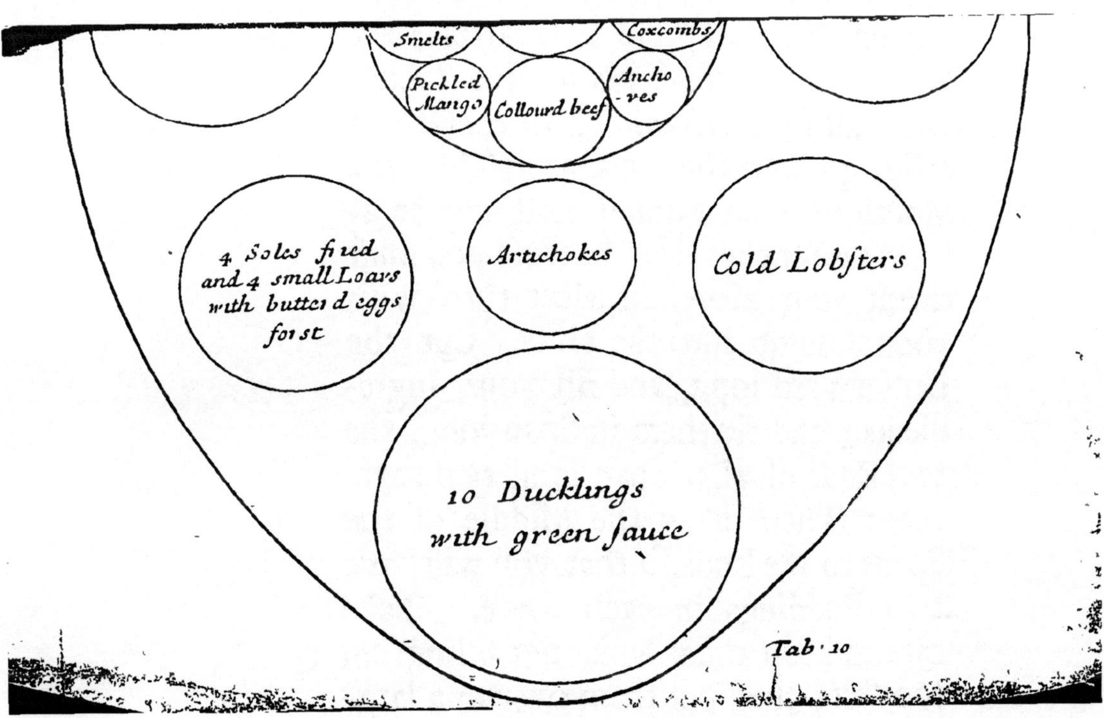
Smelts
Coxcombs
Pickled Mango
Collourd beef
Ancho-ves
4 Soles fried and 4 small Loavs with butterd eggs forst
Artichokes
Cold Lobsters
10 Ducklings with green sauce
Tab. 10

half a Nutmeg, two or three Spoonfuls of Roſe-Water, a Quarter of a Pound of Almonds, beaten as fine as Paſte in a Marble Mortar, a little Salt, mix all your Ingredients very fine together; Then have ſmall Ox Guts, or Hog's Guts, very well clean'd, and the Inſides turn'd out. Then make a ſmall Funnel that will hold a Quarter of a Pint, with a Tail about five Inches long, all of a Wideneſs, ſo that it can eaſily go into the Guts aforeſaid; the Mouth of your Funnel muſt not be above two Inches deep, becauſe you muſt thruſt your aforeſaid Meat thro' with your Thumb into the Guts. Cut the Guts a Yard long, and fill your Ingredients; and tie them in Span-long, the two Ends of that Span-long ty'd together: Then tie in the Middle of the Spans to the Ends, ſo that you will have two Puddings in each Piece. Take care to keep them lank, not filling 'em too full; then put them over in a large Braſs-Diſh of Water, and boil them gently a Quarter of an Hour, turning them with your Skimmer that the Mar-

row

row riſe not to one Side; then take them out, and lay them on a Cullender till cold, turn them in the cooling. In the Winter they will keep a Week or more, but in the Summer not above three or four days; Therefore, take care to make your Quantity according to your Diſcretion or Occaſion. About an Hour before you have Occaſion for them, place them in a Sawce-pan, and a little Butter, put them over the Fire till they fry as yellow as Gold, when one Side is yellow turn the other down, or you may put them in the Mouth of an Oven. When you ſerve, cut them aſunder. They are proper for a little Diſh or Plate for ſecond Courſe, or to garniſh a boil'd Pudding, or Fricaſſee of Chickens for the firſt Courſe. *So ſerve it.*

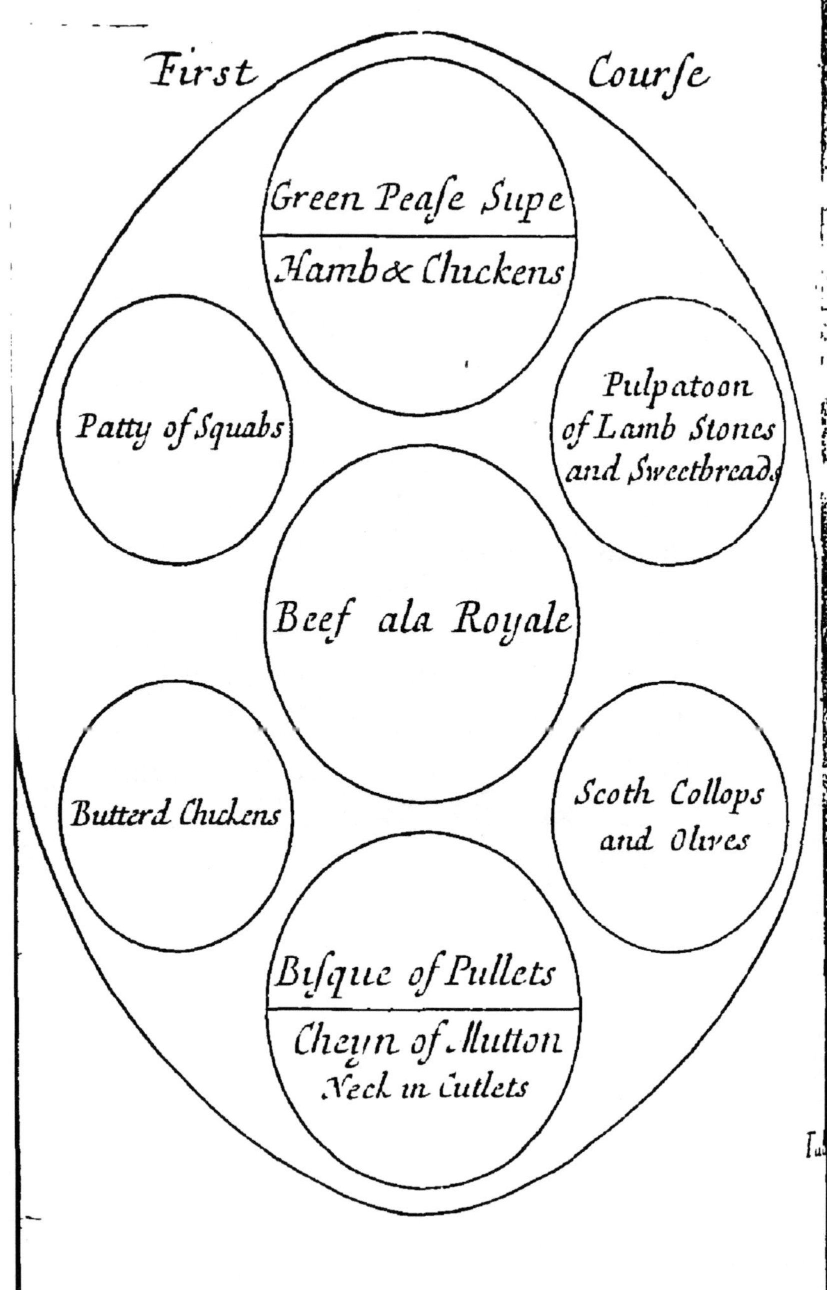
First Course
Green Peaſe Supe
Hamb & Chickens
Patty of Squabs
Pulpatoon of Lamb Stones and Sweetbreads
Beef ala Royale
Butterd Chickens
Scoth Collops and Olives
Biſque of Pullets
Cheyn of Mutton Neck in Cutlets

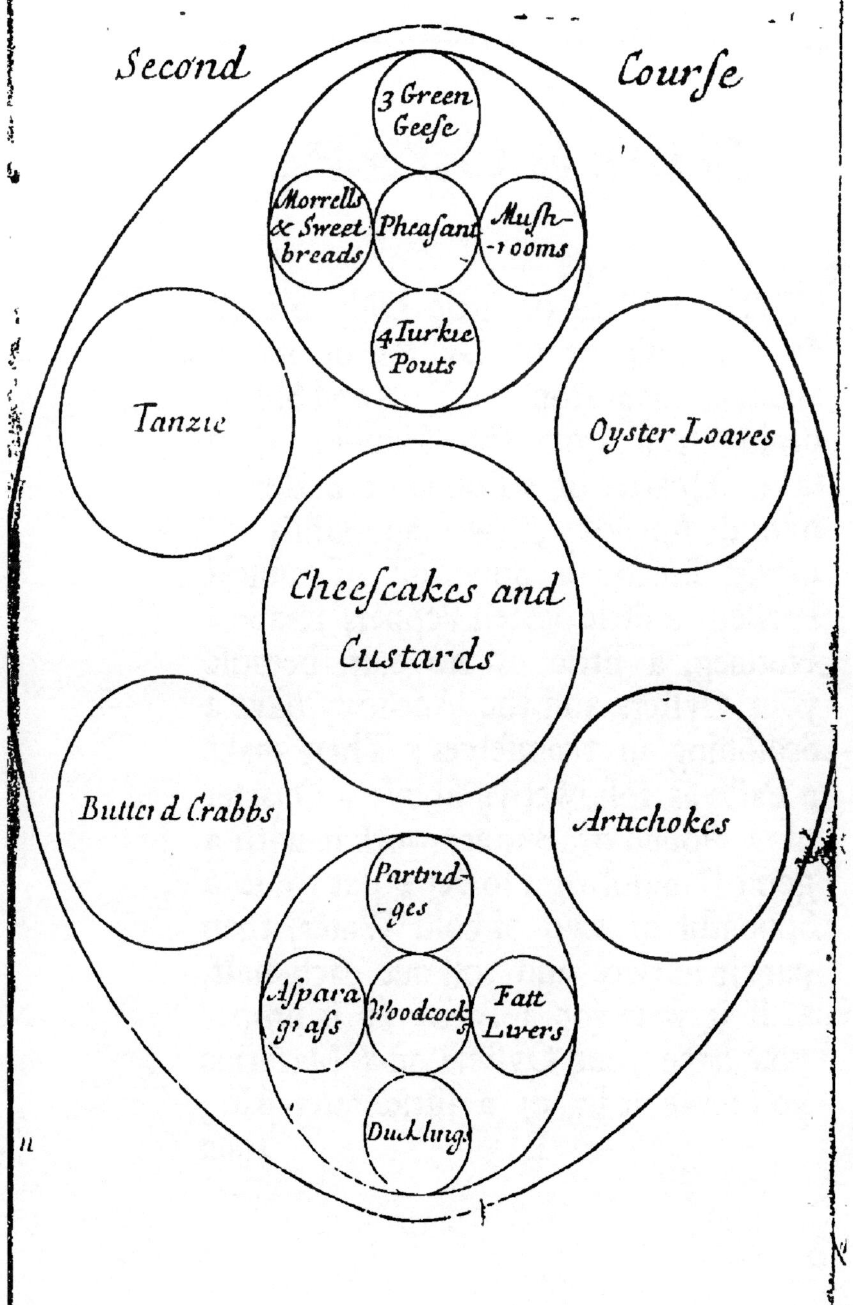

Second Course
3 Green Geese
Morrells & Sweet breads
Pheasant
Mush-rooms
4 Turkie Pouts
Tanzie
Oyster Loaves
Cheescakes and Custards
Butter'd Crabbs
Artichokes
Partrid-ges
Asparagrass
Woodcocks
Fatt Livers
Ducklings

To make an Oyſter-Pie.

FOR a Plate or little Diſh, blanch off a Quart of Oyſters or more, and take them from the Tails and Shells, drain them from the Liquor; then take a Quarter of a Pound of Butter, a minc'd Anchovy, two Spoonfuls of grated Bread, a Spoonful of minc'd Parſley, a little beaten Pepper, ſcrape a Nutmeg, a little or no Salt, becauſe your Oyſters and the Anchovy have a Seaſoning in themſelves: Then make a Paſte as followeth; above a Quarter of a Pound of Butter, work it with a good Handful of Flower; put to it a Spoonful or two of cold Water, then part it in two, and roll out each half, as if it were for a Tart. It is proper you bake your Oyſters on a Mazarine you ſerve it in, or a little Patty-pan;

then place on the Bottom-Paſte, half of your mix'd Butter, Anchovy, and Parſley aforeſaid. Then lay on your Oyſters, two or three thick at moſt; then put the reſt of your Butter and Parſley on the Top, and a Slice of Lemon; then wet it about with ſome of your Oyſter Liquor, ſtrewing a little beaten Pepper and Nutmeg over your Oyſters, and two Spoonfuls of your Liquor: Then cover it up as you do a Tart, only turn and cut it handſomely round, and turn the Edge of your Paſte, all round, an Inch high. Bake it three Quarters of an Hour before you have Occaſion for it; then cut up its Cover, and ſqueeze in a Lemon. Shake it gently together, and cut your Cover in Bits, and lay handſomely round it. *So ſerve it* for the firſt Courſe; or you may bake it without a Cover.

To make a Salmon-Pie.

IF you pleaſe, you may raiſe an Oval-Pie, ſix Inches high, and long, according to the Bigneſs of your Jole, or Side of Salmon; or you may make it in a Patty-pan: The Difference is only, if you raiſe it, it muſt be hot Paſte, but if you make it in a Patty-pan, it muſt be cold Paſte, as you did for your Oyſter-Pie, only your Quantity muſt be bigger; and your Bottom, or Upper-Cruſt muſt be as thick as any other Pie, (Veniſon and Beef excepted) becauſe the Salmon will take a good deal of Baking. Your Paſte being thus ready, prepare your Salmon as followeth: If it is for a rais'd Pie, keep your Jole whole, according to the Bigneſs of your Coffin; cut it with your Knife on the Outſide to the Bone, an Inch betwixt each Cut; and likewife joint your Chine-Bone, otherwife it will turn up, and throw off your Pie Cover in Baking; then take a Spoonful of beaten Pepper, half a Nutmeg, three Spoonfuls of Salt; rub all this very fine with the Side of your Knife on your Dreffer, and feafon your Salmon on both Sides, to your Difcretion; then take half a Pound of Butter, two fmall Handfuls of minc'd Parfley, a little Bit of minc'd Thyme, two minc'd Anchovies; mix all thefe together, with a little of your aforefaid Seafoning; then place half of it in the Bottom of your Pie; then place your Salmon and the other half over it; then put in three Spoonfuls of White-Wine, or Water, and clofe on your Cover, leaving a Vent in the Middle. Bake it an Hour and a Half or more, according to the Bignefs of your Salmon. When it is bak'd, cut off your Cover: If you find it is too fat, skim off fome, and if you find it is too dry, put to it a Spoonful or two of warm White-Wine, a Spoonful or two of drawn Butter, the Juice of a Lemon.

Serve

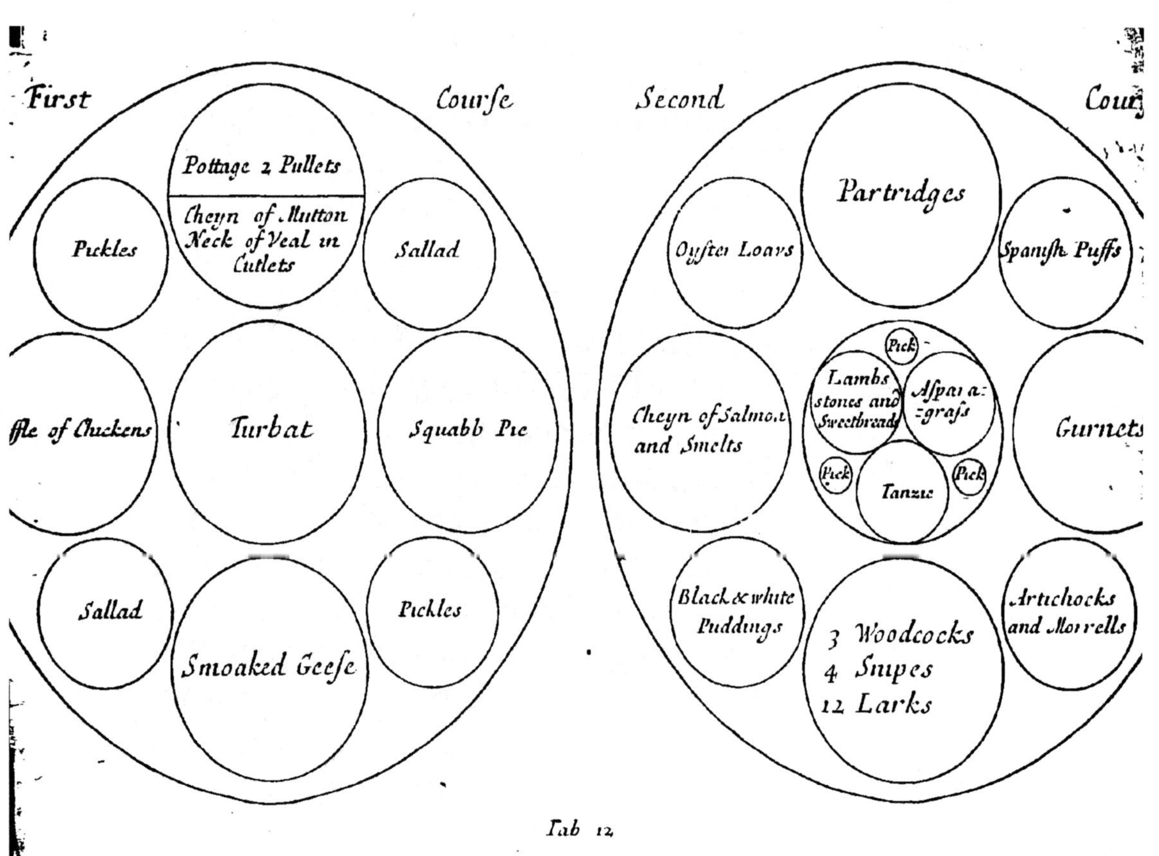
First
Course
Pottage 2 Pullets
Cheyn of Mutton Neck of Veal in Cutlets
Pickles
Sallad
ffle of Chickens
Turbat
Squabb Pie
Sallad
Smoaked Geese
Pickles
Second
Cours
Partridges
Oyster Loavs
Spanish Puffs
Cheyn of Salmon and Smelts
Pick
Lambs stones and Sweetbreads
Asparagrass
Pick
Tanzie
Pick
Gurnets
Black & white Puddings
3 Woodcocks
4 Snipes
12 Larks
Artichocks and Morrells

Tab 12

Serve it hot for the firſt Courſe, or remove without the Cover; but if you make it in a Patty-pan, cut it in Slices, as if it were to broil, or rather thicker, and lay it round the Pan on the Bottom-Cruſt; but you muſt not lay one Slice on the Top of another, and ſeaſon it, and order it, as you did for your Pie aforeſaid, only it will not take ſo much Baking by an Hour, and ſerve it without a Cover, ſhake it with the Juice of a Lemon.

To make a Salt-Fiſh-Pie.

TAKE a Side of Salt-Fiſh, or leſs, according to the Bigneſs of your Diſh, and water it well over Night; next Morning, put it over a large Pan of Water, and boil it till it is fit to eat; then throw it out in cold Water, and drain it on a Cullender, and place it with its Back to your Kitchen Table, and take all your white Fiſh clean from the Skin and Bones, ſearching the Bones nicely out with your Fingers; then mince it pretty ſmall with your Mincing-Knife. You muſt ſave a ſquare Bit of your Salt-Fiſh, as big as your Hand, whole, with the Skin on: Then take the Crum of two French Rolls cut in Slices, and boil'd up with a Pint of Cream, and a Pint of Milk; break your Bread very ſmall with a Spoon, and put to it your minc'd Salt-Fiſh, a Pound of Butter, two Spoonfuls of fine minc'd Parſley, grate in half a Nutmeg, ſome beaten Pepper, no Salt, except you find your Salt-Fiſh too freſh with the watering and boiling; if you find it too ſalt after you have minc'd it, you may put it into a Quart of cold Milk, and let it lie an Hour, then throw it into a Cullender, and ſqueeze it well from the Milk, and ſo ſtirr it over the Fire with your Ingredients aforeſaid; when you find it is of a good Taſte and good Thickneſs, ſpread it on a Diſh till it is cold. At the ſame time,

prepare

prepare a rais'd Pie or Patty-pan, as you did for your Salmon-Pie aforesaid. When it is cold, place it in with your square Piece of Salt-Fish on the Top, then cover it up as you do another Pie. If a rais'd Pie, bake it two Hours, if in a Patty-pan, one Hour. When bak'd, cut up your Cover: If there is any Oil, skim it off with your Spoon, then throw over six hard Eggs, minc'd small, and pour over it some drawn Butter, and shake it together. If you see it inclines to be oily, pour round it a little hot Milk, shake it together, and *serve it hot*. You may make a Ling or Stock-Fish Pie the same way, only instead of taking Yolks and Whites for the Salt-Fish Pie, you must take nothing but Yolks for these.

To make a Patty *of* Mushrooms.

YOur Mushrooms being fresh-gather'd, well pick'd and wash'd, put them in a Sawce-pan with a Quarter of a Pound of Butter, a little minc'd Parsley, a little Pepper and Salt, a little Slice of Bacon, stuck with four Cloves, a whole Onion; cover it up close, and stew them over the Fire, shake on them a Dust of Flower, giving them a Shake now and then as they stew, that they burn not; when their own Liquor comes to be as thick about 'em as a good Cream, throw out the whole Onion and Bacon, and set them to cool; then sheet a little Tart-pan, the Bigness of your Plate, with good fine Paste, such as you use for Tarts; let it be as thick as a Halfpenny, then pour on your cold Mushrooms

rooms, and cover it with another Sheet of Paſte, and bake it three Quarters of an Hour before you want it. Cut off your Cover, and ſqueeze in half a Lemon, ſhake it together, *and ſo ſerve it.* Or you may bake it without a Cover, but then you muſt throw over your Muſhrooms, a little brown Raſpings of a *French* Roll; when it is bak'd, ſqueeze over half a Lemon. *So ſerve it.* Your Muſhrooms being prepar'd as aforeſaid, you may likewiſe put them into Patty-pans, to garniſh a Fricaſſee of Chickens; or any Ragoo of Beef, Mutton, or Veal. Your Muſhroom Patty aforeſaid, is proper for ſecond Courſe.

To make a Lobſter-Patty.

YOur Lobſters being boil'd and cut in little Pieces, take the ſmall Claws and the Spawn, and pound them in a marble Mortar; Then put to them a Ladleful of Gravy or Broth, with a little of the upper Cruſt of a *French* Roll, when it is boil'd, ſtrain it thro' a Strainer or Sieve, to the Thickneſs of a Cream, and put half of it to your Lobſters, and ſave the other Half to ſawce them with, after they are bak'd, and put to your Lobſters the Bigneſs of an Egg of Butter, a little Pepper and Salt, ſqueeze a Lemon, put in half a minc'd Anchovy, warm this over the Fire, juſt ſo much as melts the Butter; then ſet it to cool, and ſheet your Patty-pan for a Plate or Diſh, as you did for your Muſhrooms aforeſaid. Then put in your Lobſters,

and

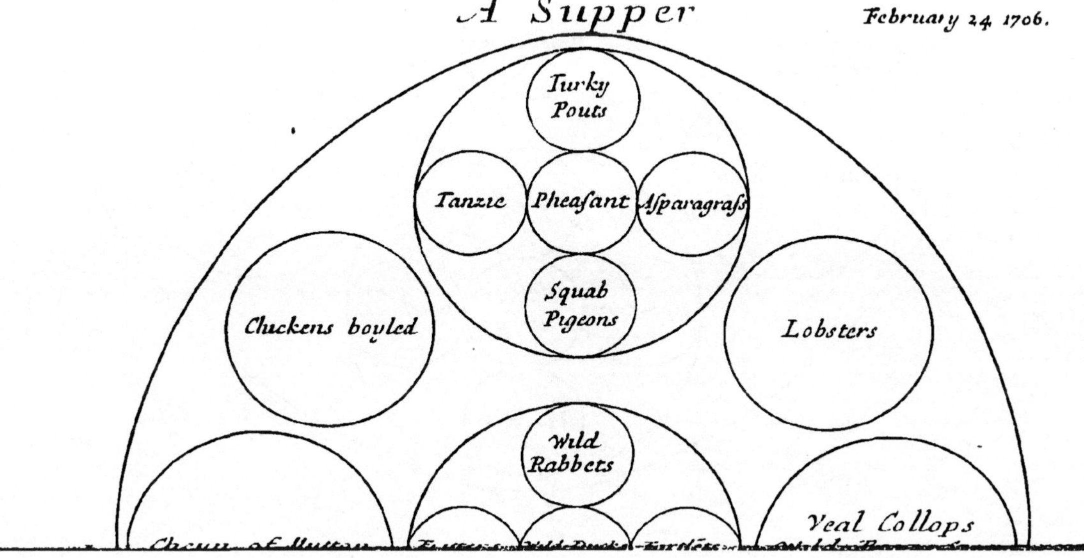
A Supper
February 24 1706.
Turky Pouts
Tanzie
Pheasant
Asparagrass
Squab Pigeons
Chickens boyled
Lobsters
Wild Rabbets
Veal Collops

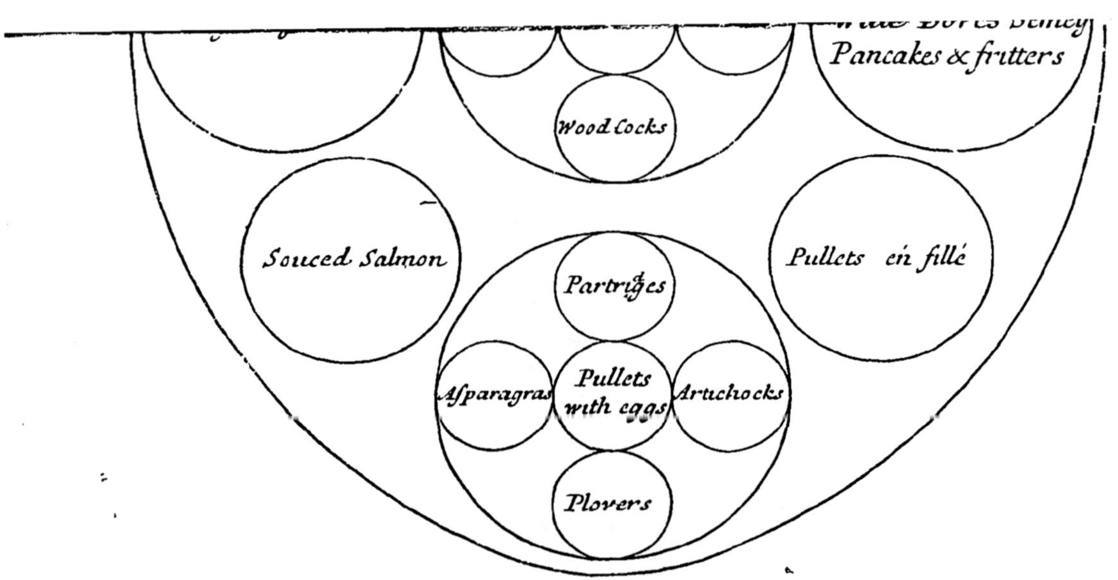
Pancakes & fritters
Wood Cocks
Souced Salmon
Pullets en fillé
Partriges
Asparagras
Pullets with eggs
Artichocks
Plovers

and cover it with a Paſte: Bake it three Quarters of an Hour before you want it; then cut up your Cover, and draw up the other Half of your Sawce aforeſaid with a little Butter, to the Thickneſs of a Cream, and pour it over your Patty, with a little ſqueez'd Lemon; cut your Cover in two, and lay it on the Top, two Inches diſtant, that they may ſee what is under. You may do Crawfiſh, Shrimps, or Prawns, the ſame Way; and they are all proper for Plates or little Diſhes, for ſecond Courſe, to the Bigneſs of your Quantity.

Pullets *in Bladders with* Oyſters.

TAKE your Pullets, and raiſe up the Skin for your Ingredients to force them withal. Take Cheſnuts, a Quart of Oyſters, hard Eggs, and Marrow, all well

well ſeaſon'd together, and then put this into your Fowl in the Skin, and ſome in the Belly: Take Bladders, and clean them very well, put your Pullets in the Bladders, and then tie them up. You may take out the Fleſh of the Pullets, and make a Forc'd-Meat of it, and force it in the Pullets again, as many Pullets as will ſerve your Diſh. For Sawce to pour over them, make a Fricaſſee of Oyſters, garniſh'd with Petit-Pattys, and haſh'd Pullets. For to bind your Ingredients, take raw Yolks of Eggs, and ſome grated Bread. They will take two Hours and a half boiling.

To make a Marrow-Tart.

TAKE the Yolks of hard Eggs, and mince them with Pippins, and the Marrow cut in ſmall Dices; mix all with Sugar, Cinnamon, and Cordicitron,

tron, and Orange-Peel minc'd very ſmall, a little Salt, the Juice of a Lemon: Mix all together, and fill up your Tart-Patty-pans with it.

To make Fine Cuſtards.

TAKE a Quart of Cream, and boil with whole Spice, then put Roſe-Water, with the Yolks of ten Eggs, and five Whites; mingle them with a little Cream, and when the Cream is almoſt cold, put the Eggs into it, and ſtir it very well; then fill up your Cuſtards and bake them. *Serve them with* French *Confits to them.*

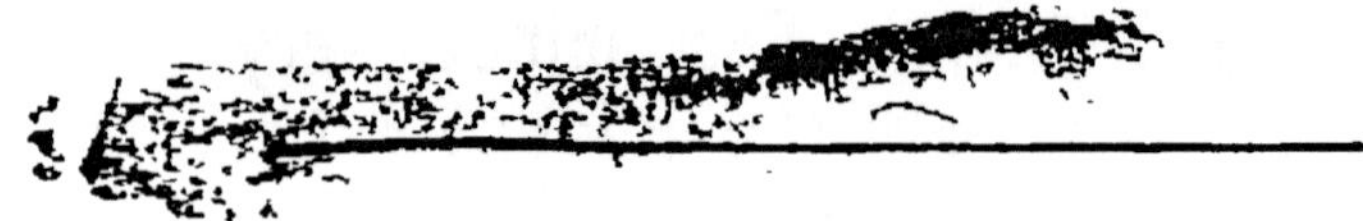

To make an Almond-Tart.

RAISE an excellent good Paſte, ſix Corners, and an Inch deep, and take ſome blanch'd Almonds, very finely beaten with Roſe-Water; take a Pound of Sugar to a Pound of Almonds, ſome grated Bread, Nutmeg, a little Cream, with ſtrain'd Spinnage, as much as will colour the Almonds green. So bake it with a gentle, hot Oven, not ſhutting the Door. Draw it, and ſtick it with Orange-Citron.

To

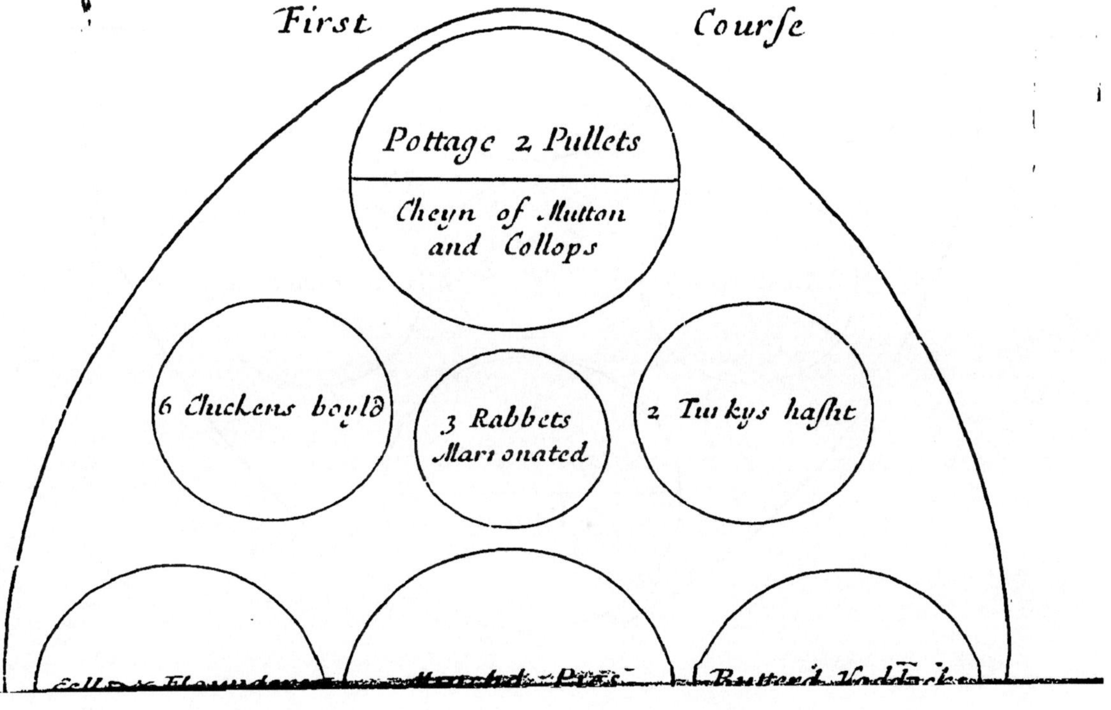

First Course
Pottage 2 Pullets
Cheyn of Mutton and Collops
6 Chickens boyld
3 Rabbets Marionated
2 Turkys hasht

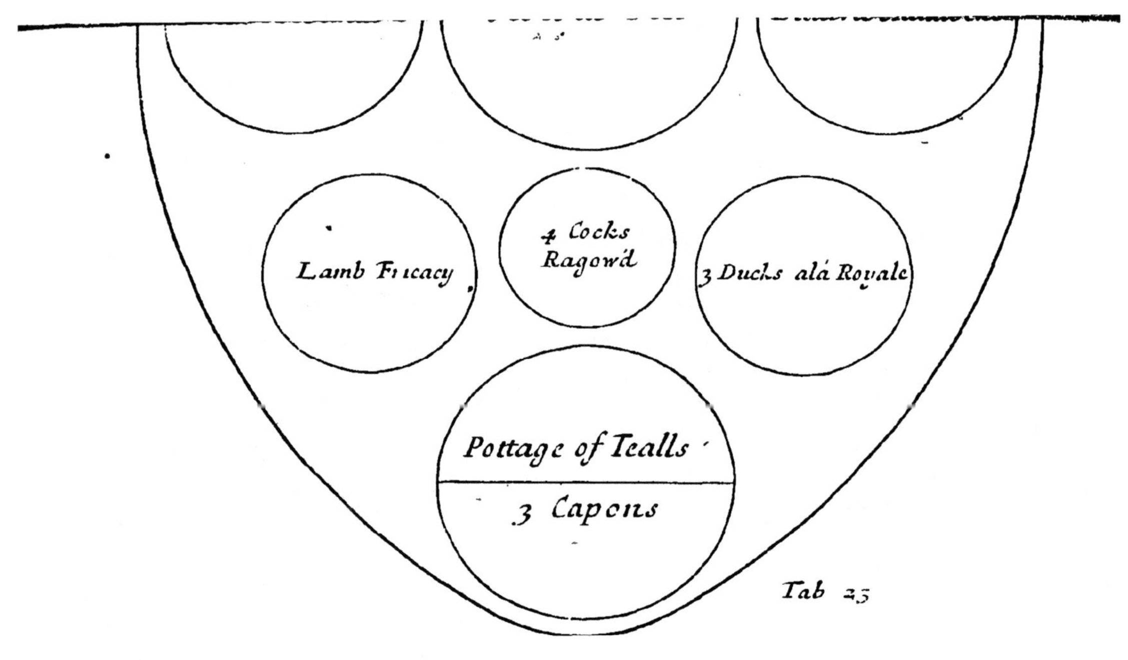
4 Cocks
Ragow'd
Lamb Fricacy
3 Ducks alá Royale
Pottage of Tealls
3 Capons
Tab 25

To stew Cabbage-Lettice.

LET your Cabbage-Lettice be clean wash'd in several Waters, take twelve for a Plate, boil them up in a Brass-Dish of Boiling-Water, half an Hour; then take them up with a Skimmer, and throw them into cold Water, squeeze the Water from them one by one, with your Hand, and place them into a little Sawce-pan; put to them a Quarter of a Pound of Butter, mix'd with a Quarter of a Spoonful of Flower, a Blade of Mace, a Bit of Bacon as big as your Thumb, stuck with six Cloves, put to them as much Veal-Broth as covers 'em quite; a little Pepper and Salt; put 'em over a clear Fire an Hour before you use 'em, or more, according to the Oldness of your Lettice; for, your Summer-Lettice will not take half the Boiling

 that

that Winter-Lettice will do; when your Broth is boil'd down as thick as a Cream about your Lettice, pour over it a little drawn Butter, and ſhake your Sawce-pan till it leers together like a Fricaſſee, but toſs it not for fear of Breaking your Lettice: Then ſlide it all out at once into your Plate or little Diſh, throwing out the Bit of Bacon and Blade of Mace. Let your Garniſhing be ſome Toaſts of Bread, or fry'd Bread about three Inches long, and two Inches broad each. This is proper for a Plate or little Diſh for Supper, or to put under boil'd Chickens for Dinner; then you may add to it a little Cream, and the Yolk of an Egg, juſt as you ſerve it. You may ſtew Sallary or Endive the ſame way, if the Place where you are, can afford it. *So ſerve it.*

To

To do Sorrel *with* Eggs.

FOR a Plate, take two Handfuls of Sorrel, well pick'd and waſh'd, put it in a Sawce-pan with a little Bit of Butter, and a little Duſt of Flower, a little Pepper and Salt, ſcrape a Nutmeg, ſtew it a Quarter of an Hour before you uſe it; pour to it two or three Spoonfuls of drawn Butter. Garniſh it with hard Eggs, cut in Quarters, one End on the Sorrel, and the other End on the Side of the Diſh, the Yolk Side up. It is propereſt for Supper, or ſecond Courſe at Dinner. *So ſerve it.*

Spinnage, *with or without* Eggs.

YOur Spinnage being well pick'd and wash'd, blanch it off a Quarter of an Hour in boiling Water, then strain it out, and squeeze it well from the Water, and mince it fine; if it is as big as a *French* Roll when it is minc'd, you may put to it half a Pint of Cream, a Quarter of a Pound of Butter, a little Pepper and Salt, scrape a Nutmeg, stew it over the Fire a Quarter of an Hour before you use it, then put it in your Plate or little Dish, and stick round about it a *French* Roll, cut it in Bits like your Finger, and fry'd brown, and lay on the Top of it six poach'd Eggs. *So serve it* for second Course, or for Supper.

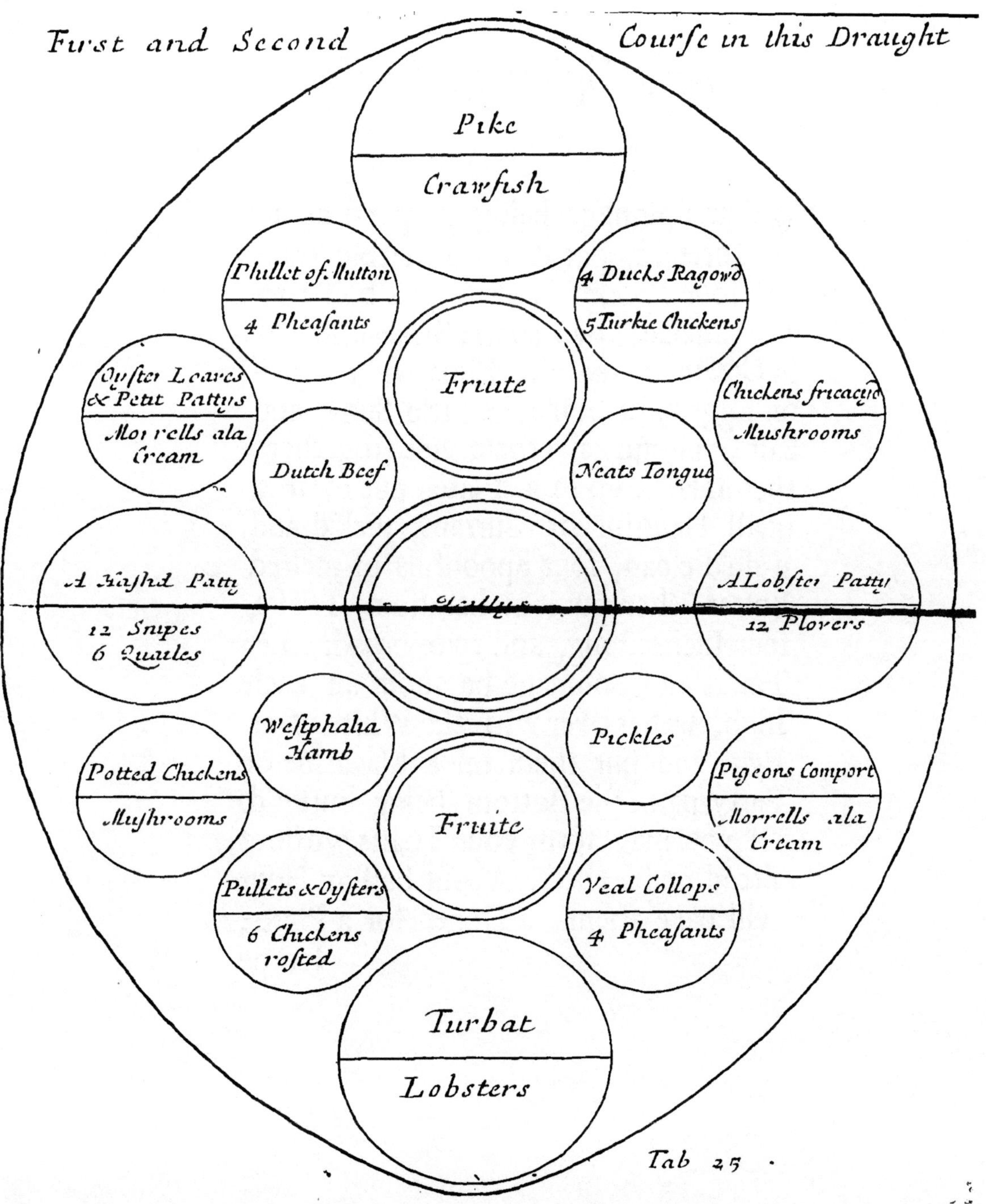
First and Second
Course in this Draught
Pike
Crawfish
Phillet of Mutton
4 Pheasants
4 Ducks Ragowd
5 Turkie Chickens
Oyster Loaves & Petit Pattys
Morrells ala Cream
Fruite
Chickens fricacyd
Mushrooms
Dutch Beef
Neats Tongue
A Hashd Patty
12 Snipes
6 Quailes
A Lobster Patty
12 Plovers
Westphalia Hamb
Pickles
Potted Chickens
Mushrooms
Pigeons Comport
Morrells ala Cream
Fruite
Pullets & Oysters
6 Chickens rosted
Veal Collops
4 Pheasants
Turbat
Lobsters
Tab 25

To make Spinnage-Toaſts.

YOur Spinnage being prepar'd as aforeſaid, put it into a Marble Mortar, four Spoonfuls of Apples boil'd to a Marmelade, two coarſe Biskets, ſoak'd in Cream, three raw Eggs, four Yolks of Eggs hard boil'd, a little Sugar and Salt; pound all theſe fine together, then take it up in a Plate, put to it a ſmall Handful of Currans, pick'd and waſh'd clean, four Spoonfuls of melted Butter; then put it on handſome Toaſts, four Inches long, and two broad. Let Toaſts and Spinnage be about an Inch high, wet it over with the White of an Egg, and put them on a Mazarine or Patty-pan, the Bottom being butter'd. Or you may form your Toaſts without Bread under them. About half an Hour will bake them, a Dozen for a Plate; ſcrape

ſcrape over a little Nutmeg, ſqueeze over half an Orange. *So ſerve it* for ſecond Courſe, or Supper.

To boil Chickens *and* Aſparagus.

FOrce the Chickens with good Force, and boil them white, cut the Aſparagus Inch long, ſo parboil it with Water, and a little Butter and Flower, and ſtrain it, and take a Sawce-pan with a little Butter and Salt, ſo let it diſſolve ſoftly, ſee that it brown not; Then add to the Aſparagus a little minc'd Parſley and Cream, a Faggot of Fennel, Nutmeg, Pepper and Salt. So ſtew it over a ſoft Fire. *So ſerve it* over your Chickens, ſqueeze in a little Lemon.

To

To make Salt-Fiſh à la Montizeur.

TAKE the Fiſh of a Carp from the Bones and Skin, mince it ſmall, put it on the Fire in a ſtewing Diſh, with a good deal of Butter, ſix whole Onions; when the Butter is melted, add the minc'd Fiſh, with Pepper and Nutmeg, ſtir it over the Fire: Your Salt-Fiſh being boil'd, take it from the Skin and Bones, and mince it as the other freſh Fiſh, with four Rolls, ſoak'd in Milk very thick, mix all theſe together, with Nutmeg and a Piece of freſh Butter; this being done, ſpread your Cod as long as your Diſh is in Bigneſs, lay on your Diſh ſome of your minc'd Fiſh. So place your whole Fiſh in the Middle of your Diſh, putting ſome of your minc'd Fiſh in about it, none on the

the Top; Put a little melted-Butter and Oysters over it, and a little grated Bread, so bake it in an Oven or Brass-Dish. Make the Sawce of Butter and Milk, and Nutmeg; bake it in the Dish you serve it in. Put the Sawce in a Porrenger to the Table, with a little over the Fish. *So serve it.*

To make a Neats-Foot Pudding.

YOur Neats-Feet being tender boil'd, take them from the Bones, and mince them very small; Half as much Sewet as Feet; mix them all together, with Sugar, Cinnamon, and Salt, a Quarter of a Pound of Citron and Orange-Peel, minc'd very fine; then break six or eight Eggs, Yolks and Whites; put them together with two Hand-

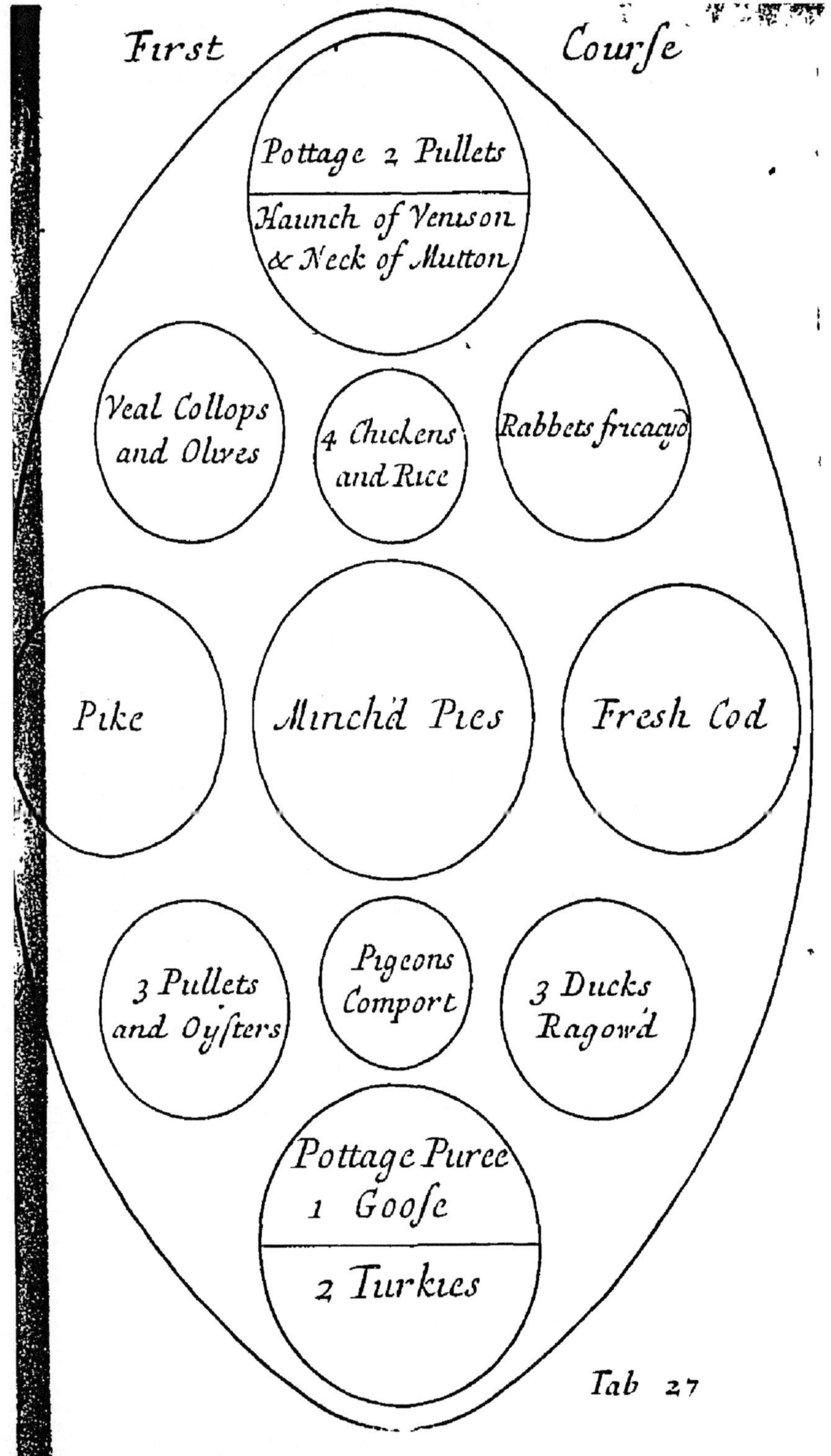
First Course
Pottage 2 Pullets
Haunch of Venison & Neck of Mutton
Veal Collops and Olives
4 Chickens and Rice
Rabbets fricacyd
Pike
Minch'd Pies
Fresh Cod
3 Pullets and Oysters
Pigeons Comport
3 Ducks Ragow'd
Pottage Puree 1 Goose
2 Turkies
Tab 27

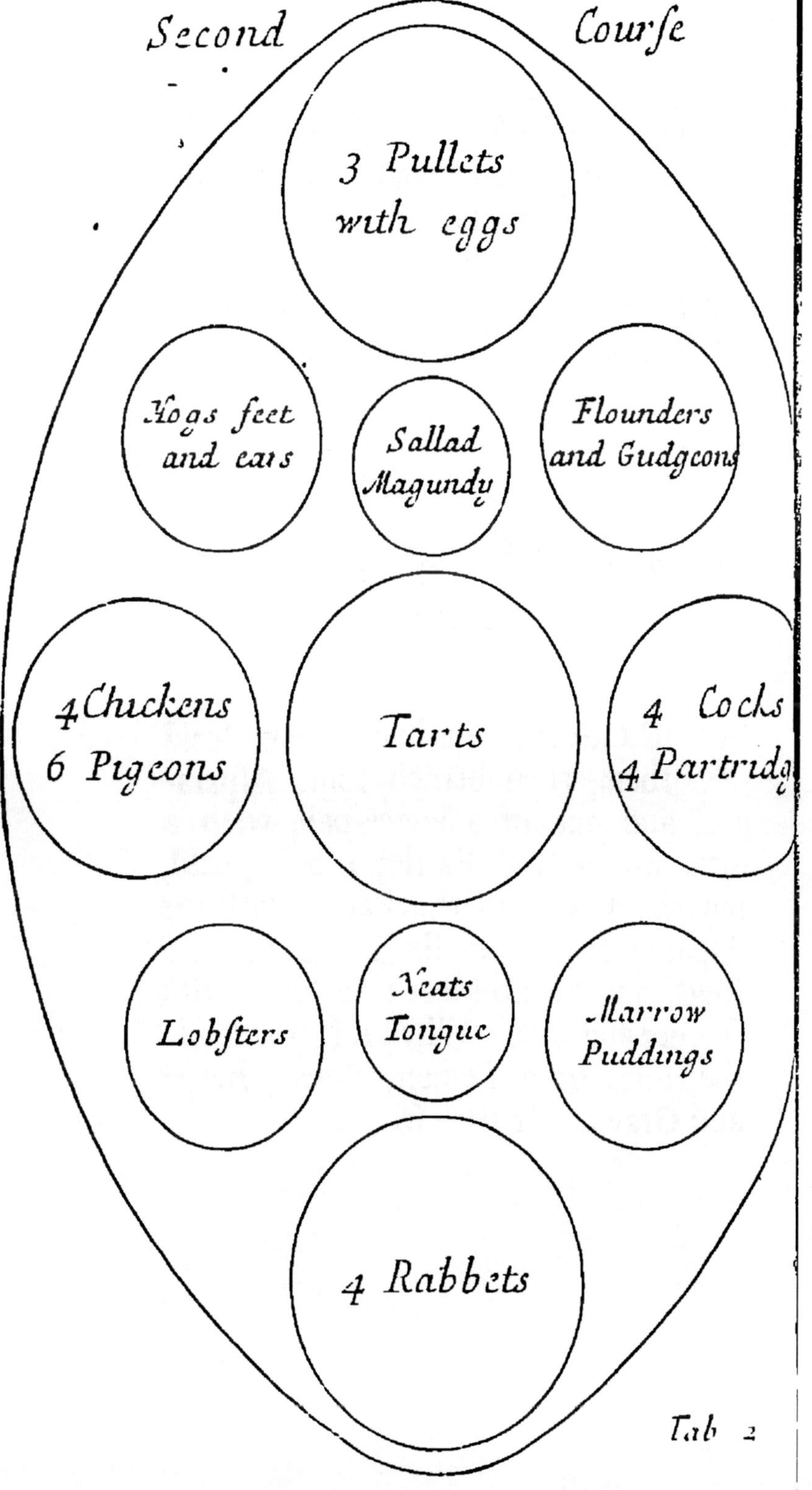
Second Course
3 Pullets with eggs
Hogs feet and ears
Sallad Magundy
Flounders and Gudgeons
4 Chickens 6 Pigeons
Tarts
4 Cocks 4 Partridg
Lobsters
Neats Tongue
Marrow Puddings
4 Rabbets
Tab 2

Handfuls of grated Bread. So mix all this together, and butter the Bag, and tie it up; boil it two Hours. *So ſerve it* with ſweet Sawce, and forget not to put ſome Currans in the Pudding.

To make a Patty *of* Calves Brains.

THE Calves Brains being clean, ſcald them, then blanch ſome Aſparagus, and put in a Sawce-pan, with a little Butter and Parſley; being cold, put the Brains in the Patty, with the Aſparagus, five or ſix Yolks of hard Eggs, and Forc'd Meat: Seaſon it with Pepper and Salt. When it is bak'd, add the Juice of a Lemon, drawn Butter and Gravy. *So ſerve it.*

To

To make Venison-Semey.

BOIL the Venison, and take it up, make a sweet Paste of a brown Loaf, grated small, mince an Orange-Peel very small, two Pound of Sugar, a Pint of White-White ; season it with Nutmeg and Salt, and mix all together with your Hand, and lap it about your Venison. So bake it an Hour. *So serve it* with a little White or *Rhenish* Wine, boil'd up with Spice and Sugar ; and Sugar over it.

To

To force Artichoaks.

BOil them, and take the Bottoms off them, and fry them with drawn Eggs, Marrow, a little Sewet, beat Pepper and Salt, grated Bread. So force your Artichoaks and Bottoms, and garnish them with it, and grated Bread. So bake them. Let your Sawce be Butter, Gravy, and Lemon. *So serve it.*

To make Chickens Chiringrate.

CUT off their Feet, and lard them, brown them off, make a Ragoo-Sawce, and stew them in it; when you are going to serve, put to your Chickens, cold Ham, slic'd. Let it stew a little with your Chickens. *So serve 'em* with your slic'd Ham about 'em.

To

To make Rosolis *of* Marrow.

CUT the Marrow in small Dices, and mince very small, and the Bigness of a Pippin, as you have Marrow, and half the Bigness of the Yolks of hard boil'd Eggs, minc'd; minc'd Cordicitron, and the Rhine of half a Lemon, very small, with Sugar, Salt, a little Milk or Cream, and Nutmeg. Mix all together, and you may make Tarts, Petit-pattys, or Rosolis of it, for your Use.

To

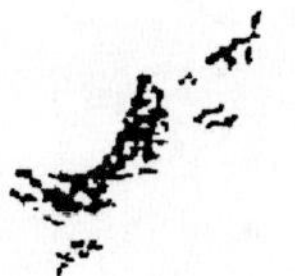

Chickens à la Braſſé.

TAKE out the Breaſts, and lard 'em and force 'em; ſo ſtew them in a Pan, and ſerve 'em. Let your Sawce be Butter, Gravy, and minc'd Parſley.

To fierce an Amlet.

TAke Kidney of Veal, mince it very ſmall, toſs it up with a little Butter and Parſley; ſeaſon it with Pepper and Salt, and the Juice of a Lemon; ſeaſon the Amlet with the ſame; make Amlets, and put the Kidneys in the Middle of the Fierce.

To make Pupton *of* Apples.

MArmelade the Apples with Sugar and Cinnamon, then add four or five Yolks of Eggs, a Handful of grated Bread, a Piece of Butter; so form it as you please: Or you may put in stew'd Pears or Cherries, according to the Season of the Year. So bake it an Hour, and turn it Upside down on a Plate for second Course.

To force Cabbage.

SCald your large Blades of your Cabbage, and make Forc'd-Meat of fat Bacon, and a Piece of Veal, a little boil'd Cabbage, the Yolks of two or three Eggs, Pepper, Salt, a little grated Bread, grated Cheeſe; ſo lap it in your Cabbage. So ſtew them in good ſtrong Broth. *Serve them* for firſt Courſe, garniſh'd with raſp'd-Cheeſe.

To boil Chickens *with* Endive.

BRown a little Butter, a little minc'd Onion, a little Anchovy and pickled Capers, mince them, and add a little Gravy. *So ſerve it* over your Chickens, to the firſt Courſe.

Veniſon à la Royale *in Blood.*

HALF roaſt it, then ſtew it, and make a Ragoo to it of Cucumers, Sweet-breads, Aſparagus. *And ſo ſerve it*, and Petits about it, and criſp Parſley.

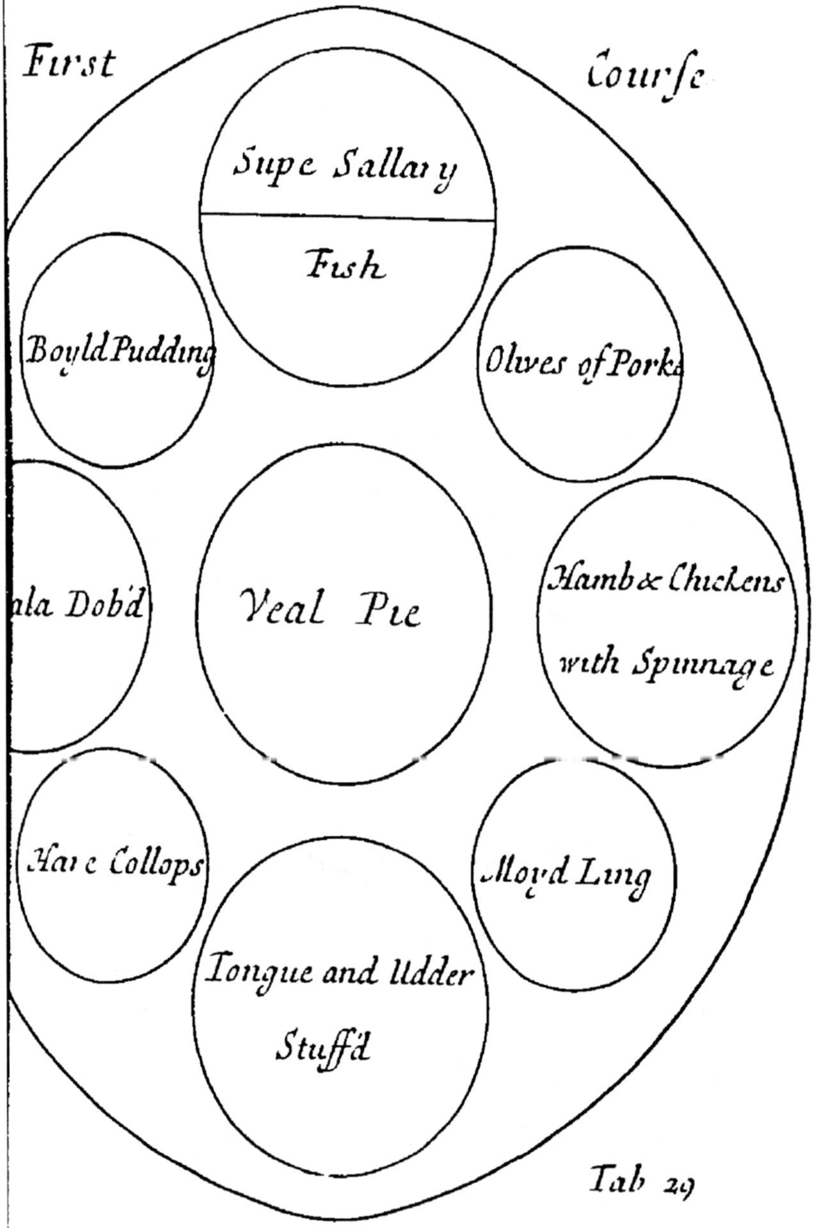

First Course

Supe Sallary

Fish

Boyld Pudding

Olives of Pork

ala Dob'd

Veal Pie

Hamb & Chickens with Spinnage

Hare Collops

Moyd Ling

Tongue and Udder Stuff'd

Tab 29

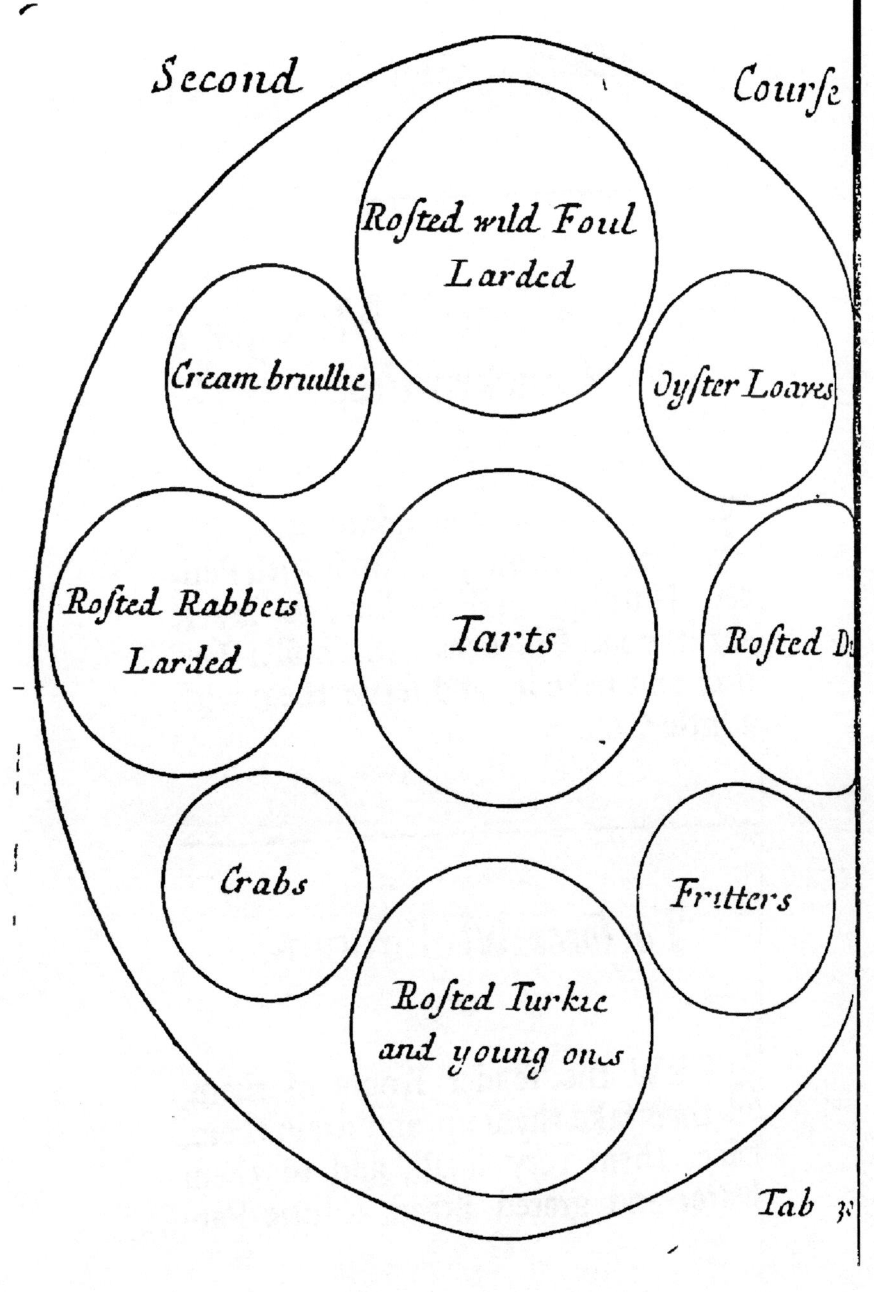
Second Course
Rosted wild Foul Larded
Cream brullie
Oyster Loaves
Rosted Rabbets Larded
Tarts
Rosted D
Crabs
Fritters
Rosted Turkie and young ones
Tab

To make a Forc'd-Meat *for a* Chicken-Pie.

TAKE Bacon and mince it, and a little Marrow; ſeaſon it with Pepper, Nutmeg, and Parſley, ſo lay it about your Chickens with boil'd Lettice, and bake it, and ſerve them with a little Caudle.

To force Muſhrooms.

STEW the tender Roots of them, then take them up and drain them, mince them very ſmall, add to them Butter and grated Bread, a little Parſley, Pepper and Salt; ſo bruiſe them well together, and force your largeſt Muſhrooms with it. Throw a little grated Bread on them, and bake them on a Petit. You may garniſh either Fricaſſee or Ragoo with them.

Civet *of* Veniſon.

BOIL the Veniſon, a Breaſt or Neck cut in Cutlets; when it is almoſt boil'd, take a Sawce-pan, and brown it in half a Pound of Butter; and as it browns, add a Quarter of a Pound of Flower, little and little, till the Brown be of a good Colour; be ſure not to burn it. Then add half a Pound of Sugar, and as much Claret as will make it the Thickneſs of a Ragoo. When you are going to ſerve it, put in the Veniſon, and toſs it three or four times, and *ſo ſerve it* with the Juice of a Lemon.

T

To make a Carrot-Pudding.

MAke it as you do another Pudding, only inftead of Sewet, put grated Carrots; And either bake it or boil it.

To make a Rice-Pudding.

BLanch the Rice in Water, then boil it in Milk and Sugar, and Cinnamon, and Salt very thick, and let it be cold, and add to it Eggs according to the Rice; but if it be to bake, half of the Whites will do; Currans and

Raisins, and a little melted Butter. Be sure if you bake or boil it, forget not Sewet, or dic'd Marrow. *So serve it.*

To make a Bread-Pudding.

TAKE a Quart of Cream, set it over the Fire to boil; Put into it a Blade or two of Mace, eight Cloves, a Bit of Cinnamon, with a little Nutmeg, Salt and Sugar; when it has boil'd, have ready the Crusts of two *French* Rolls cut in Slices and put into it, and let it stand till it is cold; then drain all the Cream that the Bread has not soak'd, and rub it thro' your Cullender, put in six Eggs, taking out two Whites; then stir it all together well, and butter your Dish, and put it in, tying it over with a Cloth and Pack-Thread. Little more than an Hour will boil it. *So serve it* with drawn Butter.

To make an Orange-Pudding.

TAke the Peel of ſix Oranges, peel'd very fine from the White, then boil them very tender, ſifting it once or twice; ſo when it is boil'd tender, beat them in a Mortar very fine, then take a Quarter of a Pound of *Naples*-Bisket, boil them up in ſome Cream, and rub it thro' your Cullender; then put your Peel to it, with the Yolks of ſix Eggs, and four Whites. Seaſon it with Nutmeg, Salt and Sugar: If there be any wanting, put in ſome Marrow, minc'd very fine. So ſheet a Pan, and bake it.

To make a Pudding-Cake.

TAke a Pound of Sewet minc'd very fine, and as much Flower, four Eggs, and a Piece of Butter; mix theſe well together; ſeaſon with Nutmeg, Sugar, Cinnamon, a little Roſe-Water and Salt. Make it into a Paſte with Cream; make it up like a Cake. So butter your Diſh, and bake it.

To do Sheeps-Rumps Sawce-Robart.

CUT your Sheeps Rumps off as near the Mutton as you can; ſix or eight will ſerve for a Plate or little Diſh, cut each in two; Put them a boiling in a Pot

Pot for the Space of three Hours, with a Spoonful of Pepper and Cloves, a good Handful of Salt, three or four Onions, a Bay-Leaf, a Sprig of Thyme, three or four Spoonfuls of Vinegar; Put in theſe Ingredients after your Pot is skim'd, only the Salt and Vinegar before; when your Rumps are very tender, and well ſeaſon'd in the Boiling, take them out, and let them drain on a Cullender, and dip them in drawn Butter, being ſcor'd on both Sides with your Knife, and turn them well in grated Bread,and broil them on a Gridiron till they are of a good Colour, then prepare your *Sawce-Robart* as followeth: Put into a Sawce-pan the Bigneſs of an Egg of Butter, when it is almoſt brown over the Fire, put to it a Handful of mix'd Onion very ſmall; fry them gently till they are brown, and throw-in half a Spoonful of Flower, fry it a little after the Flower is in, put to it a Ladleful of Gravy, a little Pepper and Salt, boil it up a Quarter of an Hour before you ſerve it, skim off the Fat juſt as you ſerve it; put to

it

it half a Spoonful of Mustard, a little Vinegar, or the Juice of half a Lemon; so pour the Sawce on the Bottom of your Dish or Plate, and lay your Rumps on the Top of it. Your Garnishing may be fry'd Parsley or Lemon, or both. *So serve it.* It is proper for first or second Course. You may do Sheep's Tongues the same way, or Hog's Feet, or Hog's Face split in two, and tender-boil'd, as you did your Rumps. This Sawce is proper also for roast Pork, or broil'd Pullets, or Pigeons, or any other Fowl; or for a roast Goose, for them that care not for Apple-Sawce.

To do Pigeon à la Tartaré *with cold Sawce.*

SInge your Pigeons, truss them as for boiling, and flat them with your Cleaver, on your Dresser, as thin as you

you can without breaking your Back or Breaſt Skin; Seaſon with Pepper, Salt, and Cloves, as if they were for a Pie; dip them in melted Butter, and drudge them with grated Bread, and broil 'em on a Gridiron half an Hour before you want 'em, turning 'em ſeveral times, and broil 'em thro'ly; or you may broil them on a Sheet of Writing-Paper well butter'd, to ſave them from the Smoke. Then provide your Sawce as followeth: Mince a Spoonful of Parſley very fine, a Shalot, or Bit of Onion, two Spoonfuls of Pickles, one Anchovy; mince all theſe very fine, apart; then ſqueeze the Juice of a Lemon, half a Spoonful of Water, ſix Spoonfuls of Oil, a little Pepper, little or no Salt, becauſe of your Anchovy and ſeaſon'd Pigeon: Mix all theſe Ingredients juſt as you ſerve it, put to it a Spoonful of Muſtard, and pour it cold on the Bottom of your Diſh or Plate, and put to your broil'd Pigeons on the Top of it ſix or eight, according to the Bigneſs of your Diſh. It is proper for firſt Courſe. *So ſerve it.*

To

To make Rhenish-Wine Cream.

PUT over the Fire, a Pint of Wine, a Stick of Cinnamon, and half a Pound of Sugar. While it is a boiling, take ſeven Yolks and Whites of Eggs, put them well together with a Whisk, till your Wine is half driven in them, and your Eggs to the Syrup; ſtring it very faſt with the Whisk till it comes to that Thickneſs that you may lift it on the Point of a Knife, but be ſure you let it not curdle; add to it the Juice of a Lemon, and Orange-Flower Water: So pour it in your Diſh, and garniſh it with Citron, Sugar, or Bisket. *So ſerve it.*

To make Forc'd Chickens Bullion Blané.

TAke the White of the Breaſts, and mince it with a little Fat Bacon boil'd, a little Marrow, a little Crum of *French* Roll, boil'd in Milk. So take the Yolks of two Eggs, the one hard-boil'd, the other raw. Mince and ſeaſon with Pepper, Salt, Nutmeg, and the Juice of a Lemon; ſo lap it up in your Chickens. So bake them. You may make Pattys of that Forc'd-Meat to garniſh your Chickens; but put neither Eggs nor Bread to your Forc'd-Meat.

To ſtew Peaſe *the* French *Way.*

TAKE Lettice, and cut them in little Bits, and three or four Onions, Slices of Bacon, a little Butter, Pepper and Salt, and toſs them over a Stove till the Lettice is hot; then add your Peaſe, and hold them ſtewing till they are tender; then add to them a little Boiling Water or good Broth: So let them ſtew ſoftly, and ſerve them with a Piece of Bacon in the Middle of the Diſh, broil'd with Parſley and grated Bread. *So ſerve it* to the firſt Couſe.

To

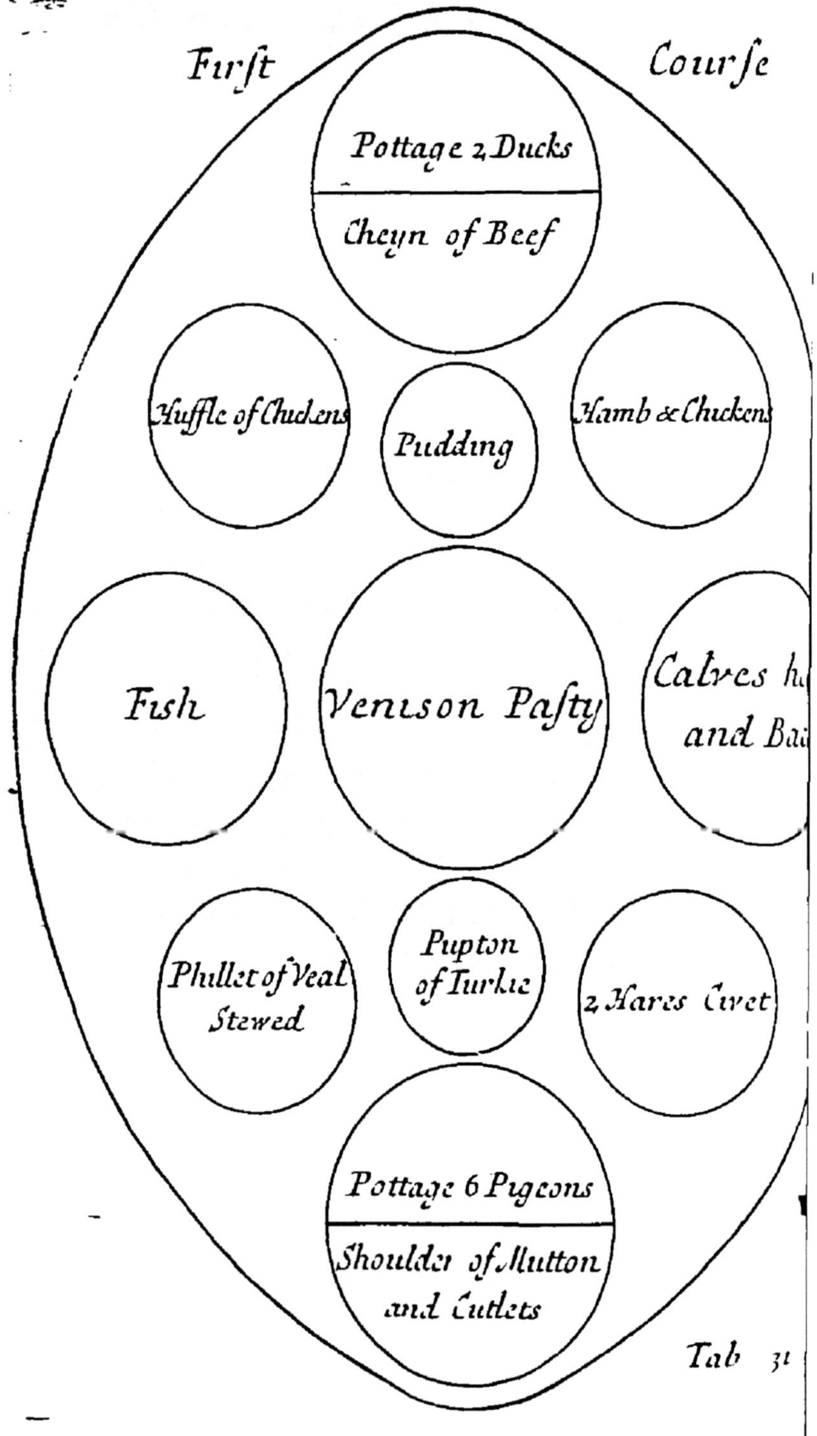
First Course
Pottage 2 Ducks
Cheyn of Beef
Huffle of Chickens
Pudding
Hamb & Chickens
Fish
Venison Pasty
Calves h
and Ba
Phillet of Veal
Stewed
Pupton
of Turkie
2 Hares Civet
Pottage 6 Pigeons
Shoulder of Mutton
and Cutlets
Tab 31

Second Course

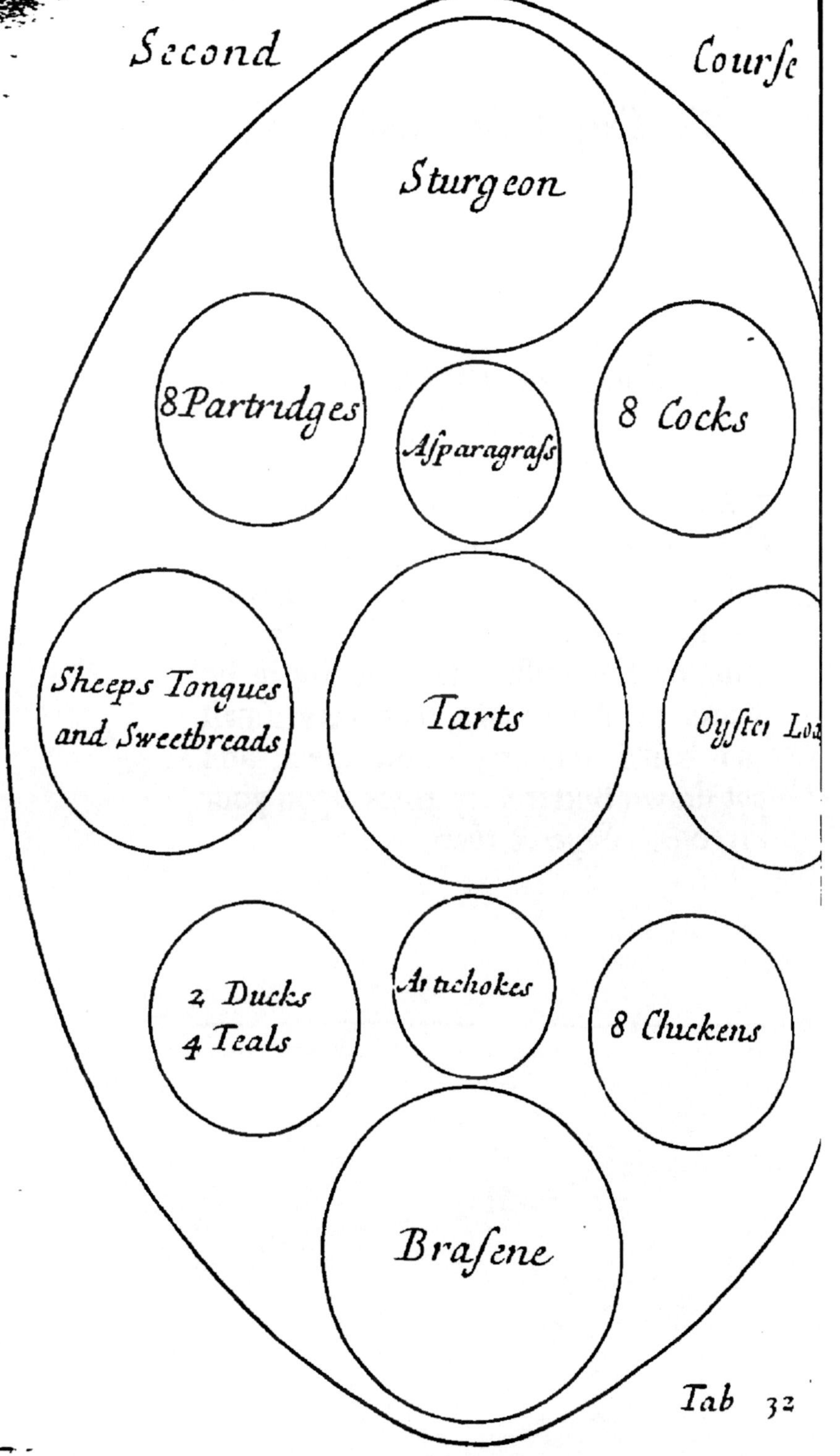

Tab 32

To force Pigeons.

MAke the Forc'd-Meat of Veal, and force the Breasts of your Pigeons, boil them, and garnish the Dish with the same Forc'd-Meat, bak'd, on the Brim of the Dish. Let the Sawce be Stucks of Artichoaks, cut very small and boil'd tender; strain them, and put drawn Butter very thick upon your Pigeons. *So serve them.*

To stew Golden Pippins *or* Apples.

CUT the Ends of your Pippins, and cut them in two, cut out the Core or Heart, place them in a Sawce-pan with the Cut Sides down, in an *English* Quart of Water, the Bigness of an Egg of Sugar, a Piece of a Rind of Lemon, cut in small Threads, about two Inches long each, as big as your Finger of Cinnamon, cover it down with a Sheet of Writing-Paper, close to your Liquor; let it simmer over a gentle Fire two hours very tender. Serve them hot or cold, for a Plate or little Dish. You must remember to pare the Skins off before you stew them. If it is a right Golden-Pippin, they will be as whole after they are stew'd as before, and as tender as Pap. Place them handsomely

ſomely on your Plate with a Spoon, lay betwixt each of them a Slice of your cut Lemon-Peel, pour over as much of your Syrup as your Plate will gently hold, ſcrape a little Sugar round. *So ſerve it.* It is proper for ſecond Courſe or Supper.

To make Black-Caps.

TAke twelve good Pippins, and cut them in two, cut out the Cores, place them on a Mazarine or Patty-pan with the Skin on, and Cut-ſide down; Put to them four Spoonfuls of Water, ſcrape over them ſome Loaf-Sugar; clap them into a pretty hot Oven, or under a Baking-Cover, till the Skins are burnt black a little in the Middle-part, and themſelves tender, which will be in three Quarters of an Hour, if your Oven is very hot. Take care it is not a Pewter Mazarine. So diſh them up for a little Diſh or Plate. Scrape a little Sugar over them. They are proper for ſecond Courſe for Supper. Or you may garniſh your ſtew'd Pippins aforeſaid with them. *So ſerve them.*

To make a Pippin Fraze.

PARE ſix Pippins, and cut out the Cores with a Penknife, cut them in thick Slices as for Fritters, or rather thicker, and fry them in a little Clarify'd Butter, turn them once, keep 'em as whole as you can, when tender, lay them on a Sieve with your Knife, that the Fat may run from them; and make a Batter as followeth: For a Plate, take five Eggs, keeping out two Whites, beat them up with a Handful of Flower, half a Pint of Cream, a little Salt, as big

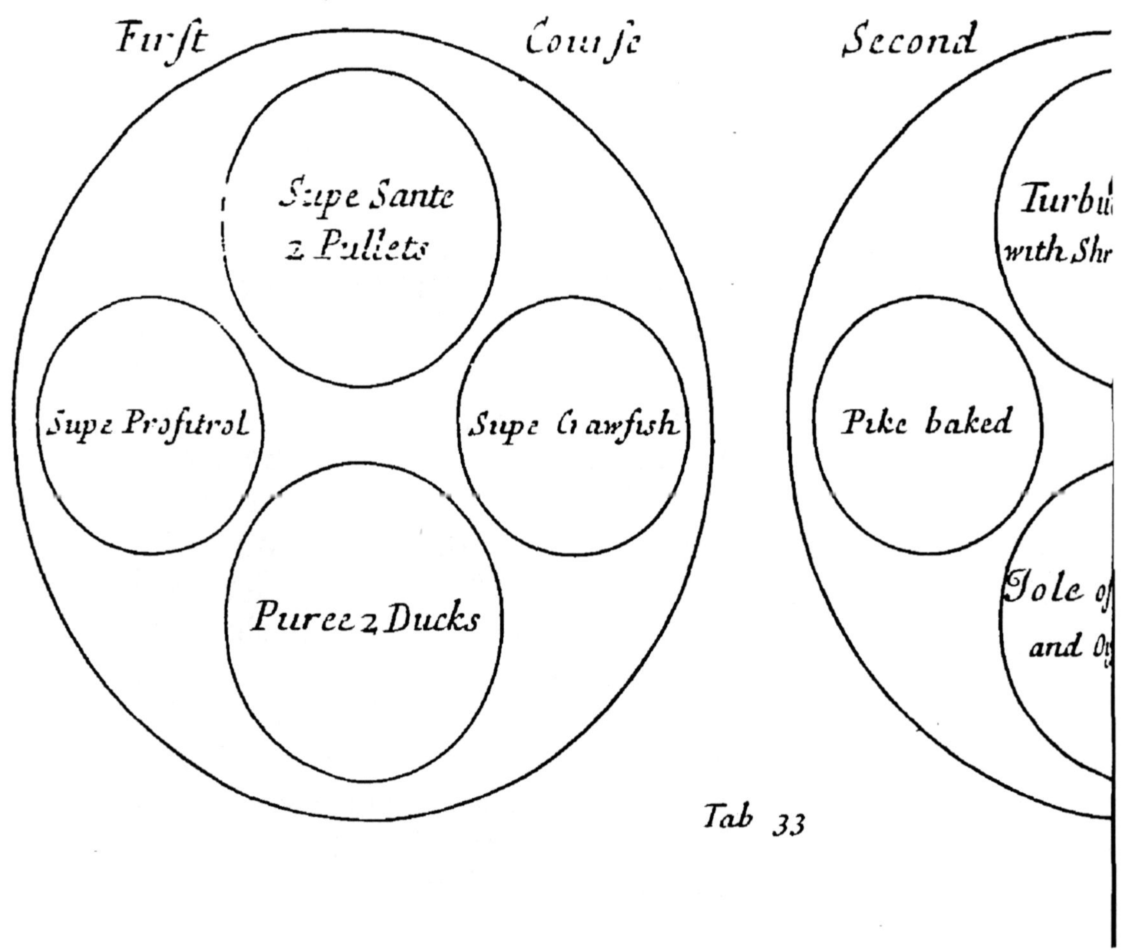
First
Course
Second
Supe Sante
2 Pullets
Supe Profitrol
Supe Crawfish
Puree 2 Ducks
Pike baked
Tab 33

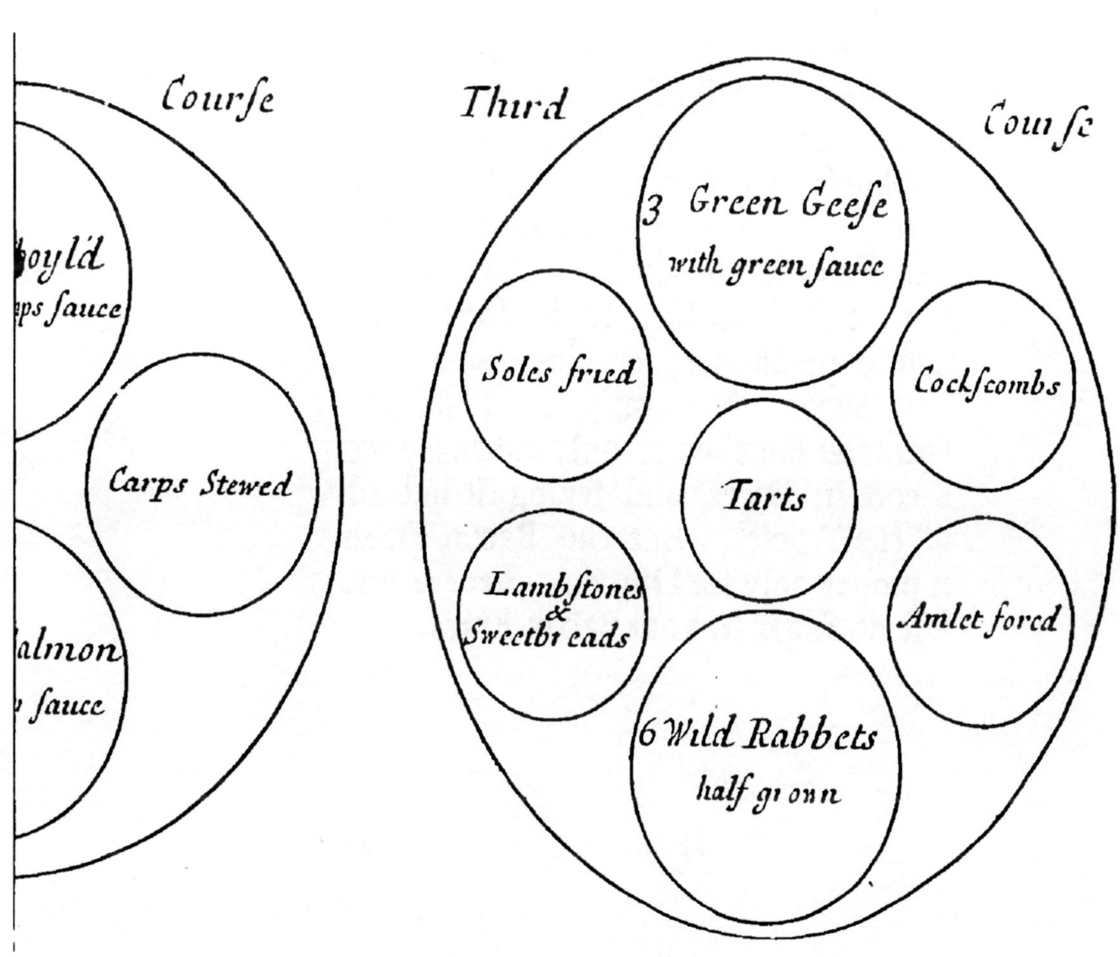
Course
boyl'd
ps ſauce
Carps Stewed
almon
ſauce
Third
Courſe
3 Green Geeſe
with green ſauce
Soles fried
Cockſcombs
Tarts
Lambſtones
&
Sweetbr eads
Amlet forcd
6 Wild Rabbets
half gr own

big as the Yolk of an Egg of Sugar, make your Batter of the Thickneſs betwixt a Fritter and a Pancake, and put into it as big as half an Egg of Butter, and put it over the Fire; then pour in half your Batter; when it is a little baked, place your fry'd Apples handſomely on it thick all over, then pour over them the reſt of your Batter; keep doing ſoftly till your Batter is of the Thickneſs that you can turn it with a Plate; then turn it once or twice till your Paſte is thro'ly bak'd, and ſerve it on a Plate or little Diſh, for ſecond Courſe or Supper, ſcraping over it a little Sugar. You may do a Bacon-Fraze the ſame way, only cutting your Bacon in Dices, and frying it inſtead of the Apples. But the Bacon-Fraze is proper only for Dinner. *Serve it hot.* Uſe no Sugar to your Bacon-Fraze.

To make Sallad-Magundy.

TAKE two or three Cabbage-Lettice, or *Roman* Lettice, being clean waſh'd, ſwing them from the Water, begin at the open End, and cut them croſs ways as fine as a Thread, and lay a Bed of it on the Bottom of your Plate or little Diſh, Inch thick; then have two Chickens or Pullets roaſted off cold, and cut the Fleſh off the Breaſts and Wings in Slices, three Inches long, as thin as a Knife, and a Quarter of an Inch broad; ſo lay it all round on the Top of your Lettice, the one End out to the Brim of your Plate, the other End to the Middle. Take ſix Anchovies from the Bones, cut each in eight Slices, and lay all round betwixt your Fowl; then take the lean Meat of the Legs of your Pullets or Chickens

cut

cut in ſmall Dices, the Yolks of four hard Eggs minc'd with it, a little minc'd Parſley, a little minc'd Anchovy, a little dic'd Lemon; Make this in a round Heap in the Middle, like the Top of a Sugar-Loaf; then garniſh it with ſmall Onions, as big as Yolks of Eggs, boil'd in a good Quantity of Water, very white and tender; put the biggeſt of your Onions on the Middle of your minc'd Meat, on the Top of your Sallad, the reſt all round the Brim of your Plate, as thick as they can lie one by another. *So ſerve it* for firſt or ſecond Courſe. Juſt as you ſend it up, beat up ſome Oil and Vinegar, Pepper, and Salt, and pour all over it. But this is commonly done at Table. You may garniſh this Sallad with ſome Grapes, juſt ſcalded, or with *French* Beans blanch'd off, or Station-Flowers; or you may put under it, inſtead of Lettice, a little ſmall Sallading.

To make Cream-Toasts, *or* Pain Perdu.

TAKE two *French* Rolls, or more, according to the Bigneſs of your Diſh, and cut them in thick Slices, as thick as your Finger, Crum and Cruſt thro', lay them on a Silver or Braſs-Diſh, put to them a Pint of Cream, half a Pint of Milk; ſtrew over them beaten Cinnamon and Sugar, turn them frequently till they are tender ſoak'd, ſo as you can turn them without breaking; ſo take them with a Slice or Skimmer from your Cream; break four or five raw Eggs, turn your Slices of Bread in the Eggs, and fry them in Clarify'd Butter; make them of a good brown Colour, not black; take care of Burning them in frying; Scrape a little Sugar round them, have a

care

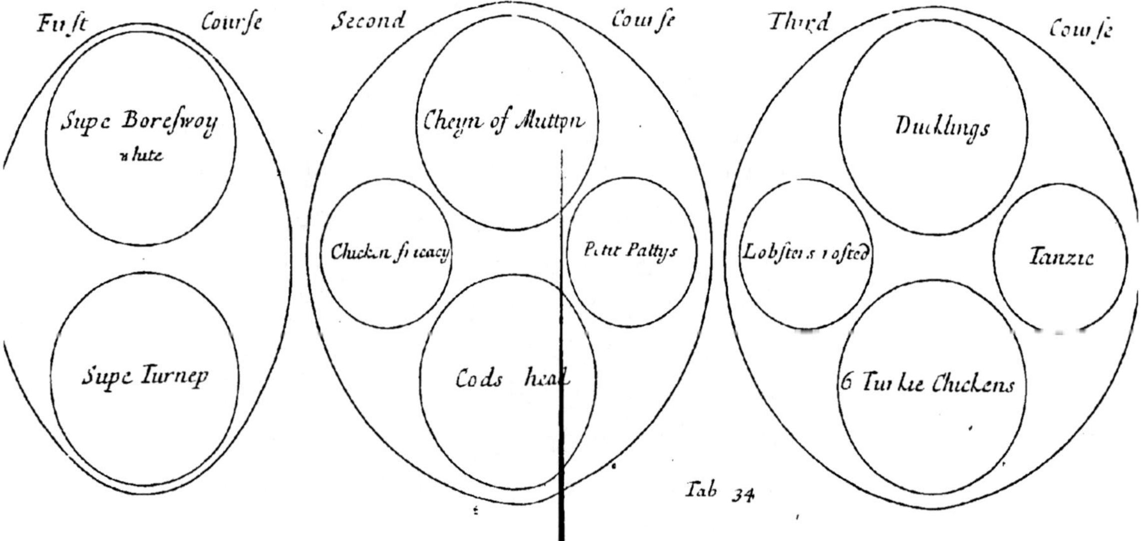

Fi st Course
Supe Boreswoy
white
Supe Turnep
Second Course
Cheyn of Mutton
Chicken fricacy
Petit Pattys
Cods head
Third Course
Ducklings
Lobsters rosted
Tanzie
6 Turkie Chickens
Tab 34

care you make them not too ſweet. You may *ſerve them hot* for ſecond Courſe, being well drain'd from your Butter in which you fry'd them; but they are moſt proper for a Plate or little Diſh for Supper.

To make Fry'd-Cream.

PUT over the Fire in a Sawce-pan a Pint of Cream, half a Pint of Milk, a Piece of Sugar, a Piece of Cinnamon; let it ſimmer over the Fire ſoftly, a Quarter of an Hour. In the mean time, break eight Yolks, ſix Whites of Eggs in another Sawce-pan, beat them together with a wooden Spoon or Ladle, and add to them a Quarter of a Pint of Cream, a Handful or two of fine Flower, and mix all together as fine as can be; your Stick of Cinnamon being taken out, add

add to it your boiling Cream, and boil it over the Fire, ſtirring it hard for a Quarter of an Hour, add to it a little Salt, and Citron minc'd fine; being all boil'd together of a Thickneſs that you can juſt ſtir it, flower a Mazarine, and pour it out upon it, make it run a Breadth with your Hand, till it is the Thickneſs of your Thumb, ſtrew a little Flower over it; cut it out with a Knife in Squares or Diamonds, three Inches long, flower it as you cut it, and fry it in Hogs Lard, *and ſerve it hot*, with a little ſcrap'd Sugar, for ſecond Courſe or Supper.

To make Jelly.

TAke a Pound of Harts-Horn, put it in a clean Pot, with ſix Quarts of Water, and let it boil over a gentle Fire till it comes to a Jelly; if the Harts-Horn is good, you may boil two Quarts away, ſo that you will have four Quarts of Jelly; take out a little in a Spoon to cool; when you find it to hang on your Spoon, it is enough: Take care to make it a little ſtronger in the Summer than the Winter. Boil your Stock off thus, the Night before you uſe it, next Morning take it up and leave the Grounds; but you muſt remember to ſtrain it from the Harts-Horn when it is hot, then put it into a clean Braſs-Diſh, cold. If you have four Quarts of it, put to it a Bottle of *Rheniſh*-Wine, beat up the Whites of eight Eggs to a Froth, and put to it likewiſe twelve Cloves, two Blades of Mace, as big as your Finger of Cinnamon.

mon. These Ingredients being mix'd cold in a well-tinn'd Brass-Dish or little Pot, set your Stock over a clear Fire, stirring it with a clean Ladle, and pour it in as if you were cooling any thing, to mix the Whites of your Eggs well with your Jelly; so after it has boil'd up two or three Minutes, put to it the Juice of six or eight Lemons. But you must remember when you put in your Whine, to put in half a Pound of Loaf-Sugar, you may sweeten it or sharpen it according to your Discretion, and Palate of the Eater. Let it boil up two Minutes after you put in your Lemon-Juice, and when you see it finely curl'd and of a pure white Colour, have your Swan-Skin Jelly-Bag hang on a clean Dish or Sawce-pan, then pour your Jelly softly into it with your Ladle. The first Quart or two that runs thro', put it back into your Jelly-Bag softly till you find your Jelly is as clear as Rock-water. If in Winter time, you had best let your Jelly run by the Fire; for in the cold, it will be apt to stop in the Running. So you

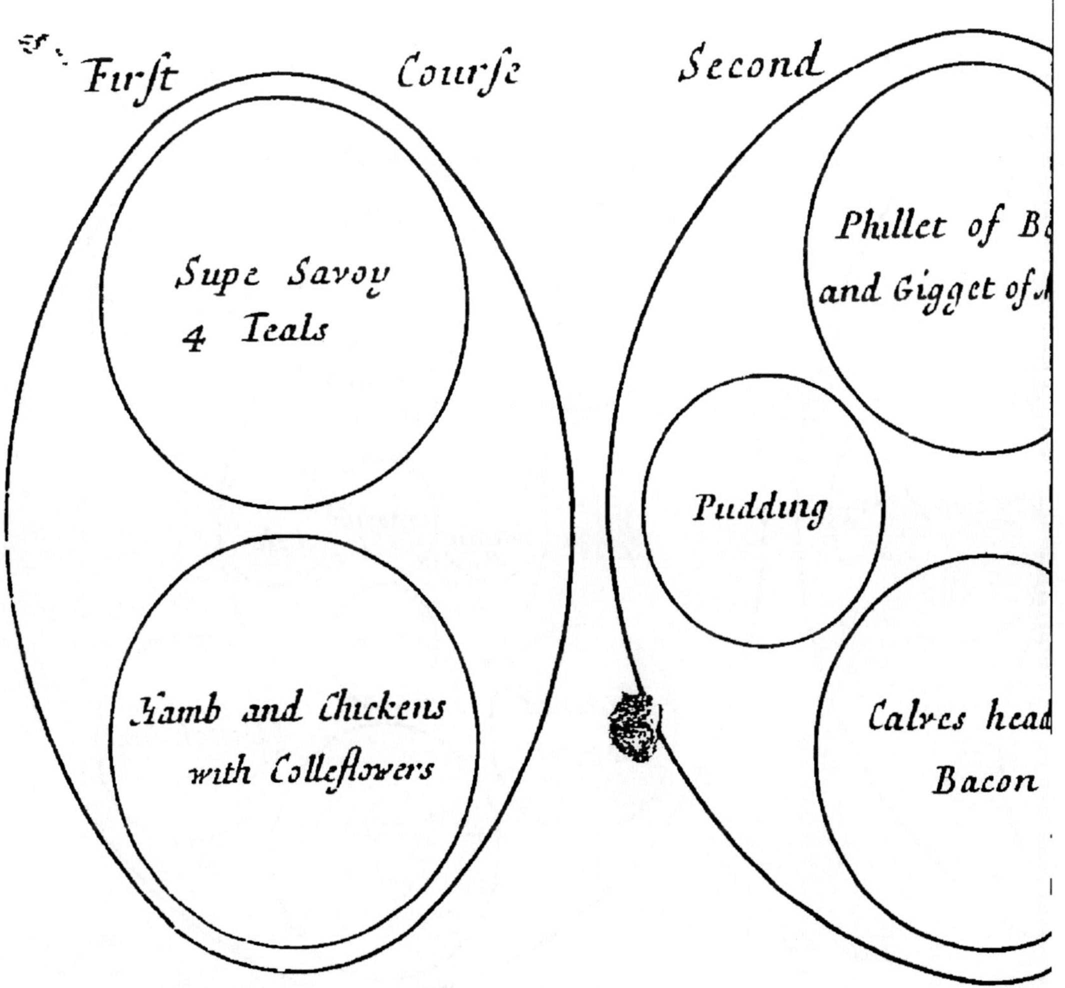
First Course Second
Supe Savoy
4 Teals
Hamb and Chickens
with Colleflowers
Phillet of B
and Gigget of M
Pudding
Calves head
Bacon

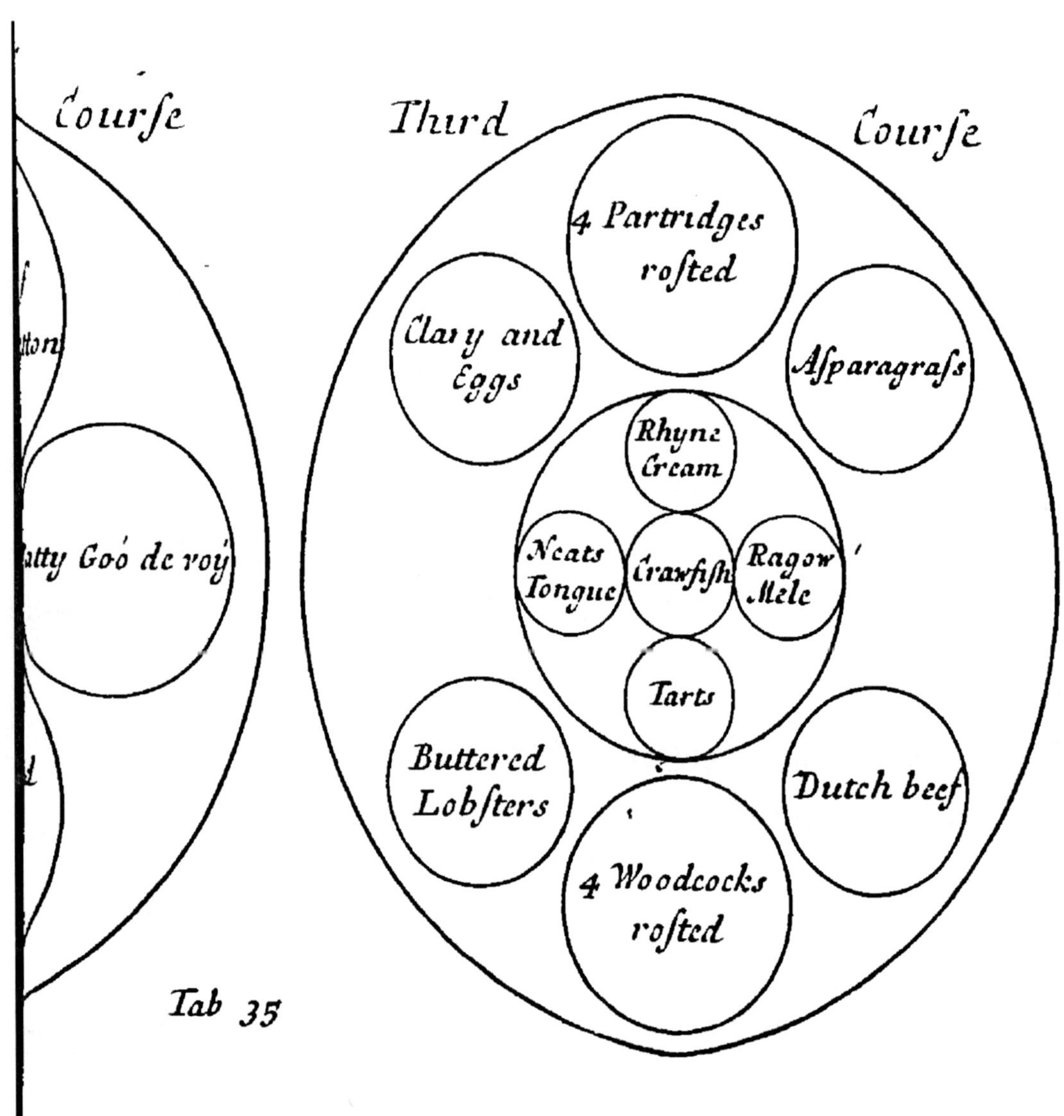
Course
Third
Course
4 Partridges
rosted
Clary and
Eggs
Asparagrass
Rhyne
Cream
Neats
Tongue
Crawfish
Ragow
Mele
Tarts
Buttered
Lobsters
Dutch beef
4 Woodcocks
rosted
tton
atty Goó de roy
Tab 35

you may fit up your Jelly-Glaſſes or *China* fit for your Uſe.

To make Blamangé.

BLanch off a Pound of Almonds in ſcalding Water, take off all the Husks, pound them as fine as Paſte in a Marble Mortar, or Stone Mortar; as you pound them, put to them, now and then, a Spoonful of your aforeſaid Jelly, to keep them from oiling; when they are very fine, put them into a clean Sawce-pan, with a Quart or three Pints of your aforeſaid Jelly; warm it over the Fire till it is ſcalding hot, breaking your Almonds well with your Jelly, with a Silver or wooden Ladle; Then take it off and ſtrain it thro' a woolen Strainer, or Table-Napkin, into a Diſh, rubbing your Almonds thro' as hard as you can with your Ladle; pour back your Jelly on your Almonds three or four times, till you find your

Bla-

Blamangé is almoſt as thick as a Cream, otherwiſe it will be apt to part when it is cold, the Almonds ſwimming on the Top, and the Jelly falling to the Bottom; and that doth not look well, and it is a Token that your Almonds were not well beat, or not often enough ſtrain'd. This done, you fit up Jelly-Glaſſes, to ſet betwixt your plain Jelly; or put it in a *China*-Bowl, for the Middle of the Diſh, or cold Plates for ſecond Courſe. Likewiſe two Glaſſes of each Sort in the Vacancies of your Plates, the White oppoſite to one another, and ſo the other. Or, with theſe two Jellies you may make a Diſh for ſecond Courſe by themſelves. I have aſſerted this, becauſe mixing the Ingredients cold for your plain Jelly aforeſaid, I think is better than putting your Eggs into your Stock after it boils. This way of mixing the Ingredients cold, is not commonly known. You may make the plain Jelly aforeſaid, in caſe of Neceſſity, of two Gang of Calves-Feet. In buying of your Harts-Horn, you muſt take care, becauſe there is a great Cheat in in it. For, ſome ſcrape Bones, inſtead of Harts-Horn; and then it will not be ſo fine, nor make ſuch a great Quantity as aforeſaid. Theſe two are proper for ſecond Courſe or Supper, and ſome uſe it for a Deſart. You may make half the Quantity with half the Ingredients, according to your Occaſion. If the Eater loves it, you may uſe a little Musk in the running of your Jelly, ty'd in a Rag, and thrown into your Jelly Bag; but moſt Quality love it plain. If you have a Mind to make any Colours, take what Quantity of your Jelly you pleaſe. For red, ſqueeze thro' a Bit of clean Cloth, a little Cocheneal: For yellow, a little Saffron. Waſh your Jelly Bag out in cold Water. Be ſure, let not Smoke come near it, and that it be very dry, when you run your Jelly, and do not ſhake your Bag as you pour it in, for it will be apt to ſtop. When you uſe your Bag, hang it on a Plate, or Spit, with the Mouth Open.

End of the Receipts.

A Bill of Fare for January.

First Course.

COllar of Brawn
Bisque of Fish
Pottage with Vermisselly
Orange Pudding, with Patties
Chine and Turkey
Lamb Pasty
Rosted Pullets with Eggs
Oyster Pye
Roasted Lamb in Joints
Grand Sallad, with Pickles.

Second Course.

Wild-Fowl of Sorts
Chine of Salmon broil'd with Smelts
Fruit of sorts
Jole of Sturgeon
Collar'd Pig
Dry'd Tongues, with salt Sallads
Marinated Fish.

I *For*

For February.

First Course.

POttage *Lorrain*
Turbot boil'd with Oyſters and Shrimps
Grand Patty
Hen-Turkeys with Eggs
Marrow Pudding
Stew'd Carps and broil'd Eels
Spring Pye
Chine of Mutton, with Pickles
Diſh of Scotch-Collops
Diſh of Sallad Magundy.

Second Course.

Fat Chickens and tame Pigeons
Aſparagus and Lupins
Tanzey and Fritters
Diſh of Fruit of ſorts
Diſh of fry'd Soles
Diſh of Tarts, Cuſtards and Cheeſecakes.

For

For March.

First Course.

DIsh of Fish of sorts
Pottage Sante
Westphalia-Ham and Pigeons
Batelio Pye
Pole of Ling
Dish of roasted Tongues and Udders
Pease Soupe
Almond Puddings of sorts
Olives of Veal alamode
Dish of Mullets boil'd.

Second Course.

Broil'd Pike
Dish of Notts, Ruffs, and Quailes
Skerret Pye
Dish of Jelleys of sorts
Dish of Fruit of sorts
Dish of Creamed Tarts.

A Bill of Fare for

For April.

First Course.

WEstphalia-Ham and Chickens
Diſh of haſh'd Carps
Biſque of Pigeons
Lumber pye
Chine of Veal
Grand Sallad
Alamode Beef
Almond Florentines
Fricaſſee of Chickens
Diſh of Cuſtards.

Second Course.

Green Geeſe and Ducklings
Butter'd Crab, with Smelts fry'd
Diſh of Sucking Rabbets
Rock of Snow and Sullebubs
Diſh of ſowc'd Mullets
Butter'd Apple-pye
March Pain.

For

For May.

First Course.

JOle of Salmon, *&c.*
Craw-fish Soupe
Dish of Sweet Puddings of Colours
Chicken-pye
Calves-Head hash'd
Chine of Mutton
Grand Sallad
Roasted Fowls aladobe
Roasted Tongues and Udders
Ragoo of Veal, *&c.*

Second Course.

Dish of young Turkeys larded, and Quails
Dish of Pease
Bisque of Shell-fish
Roasted Lobsters
Green Geese
Dish of Sweetmeats
Oringado-pye
Dish of Lemon and Chocolate Creams
Dish of collar'd Eels, with Craw-fish.

For June.

First Course.

ROasted Pike and Smelts .
Westphalia-Ham and young Fowls
Marrow Pudding
Haunch of Venison roasted
Ragoo of Lamb-stones and Sweetbreads
Fricassee of young Rabbets, *&c.*
Umble Pyes
Dish of Mullets
Roasted Fowls
Dish of Custards.

Second Course.

Dish of young Pheasants
Dish of fry'd Soles and Eels
Potato-pye
Jole of Sturgeon
Dish of Tarts and Cheesecakes
Dish of Fruit of sorts
Sullebubs.

For July.

First Course.

COck Salmon, with butter'd Lobster
Dish of Scotch-collops
Chine of Veal
Venison-pasty
Grand Sallad
Roasted Geese and Ducklings
Patty Royal
Roasted Pig larded
Stew'd Carps
Dish of Chickens boil'd with Bacon, *&c.*

Second Course.

Dish of Partridges and Quails
Dish of Lobsters and Prawns
Dish of Ducks and tame Pigeons
Dish of Jellys
Dish of Fruit
Dish of marinated Fish
Dish of Tarts of sorrs

For August.

First Course.

Westphalia-Ham and Chickens
Bisque of Fish
Haunch of Venison roasted
Venison-pasty
Roasted Fowls aladobe
Umble Pyes
White Fricassees of Chickens
Roasted Turkeys larded
Almond Florentines
Alamode Beef.

Second Course.

Dish of Pheasant and Partridges
Roasted Lobsters
Broil'd Pike
Creamed Tart
Rock of Snow and Sullebubs
Dish of Sweetmeats
Sallad-Magundy.

For

For September.

Firſt Courſe.

BOIL'D Pullets with Oyſters, Bacon, *&c.*
Biſque of Fiſh
Batelio Pie
Chine of Mutton
Diſh of Pickles
Roaſted Geeſe
Lumber Pie
Olives of Veal with Ragoo
Diſh of boil'd Pigeons with Bacon,

Second Courſe.

Diſh of Ducks and Teal
Diſh of Fry'd Soles
Butter'd Apple-Pie
Jole of Sturgeon
Diſh of Fruit
March Pain.

For

For October.

First Course.

WEstphalia Ham and Fowls
Cods-head with Shrimps and Oysters
Haunch of Doe with Udder a la Force
Minc'd Pies
Chine and Turkey
Bisque of Pigeons
Roasted Tongue and Udder
Scotch-Collops
Lumber Pie.

Second Course.

Wild Fowl of Sorts
Chine of Salmon Broil'd
Artichoak Pie
Broil'd Eel and Smelt
Sallad-Magundy
Dish of Fruit
Dish of Tarts and Custards

For November.

Firſt Courſe.

BOIL'D Fowls with Savoys, Bacon, *&c.*
Diſh of Stew'd Carps and Scollop'd Oyſters
Chine of Veal and Ragoo
Sallad and Pickles
Veniſon Paſty
Roaſted Geeſe
Calves Head haſh'd
Diſh of Gurnets
Grand Patty
Roaſted Hen-Turkey with Oyſters.

Second Courſe.

Chine of Salmon and Smelts
Wild Fowl of Sorts
Potato Pie
Slic'd Tongues with Pickles
Diſh of Jellies
Diſh of Fruit
Quince Pie.

A Bill of Fare &c.

For December.

First Course.

WEstphalia Ham and Fowls
Pottage with Teal
Turbot with Shrimps and Oysters
Marrow Pudding
Chine of Bacon and Turky
Batelio Pie
Roasted Tongue and Udder, and Hare
Pullets and Oysters,Sawsages *&c.*
Minc'd Pies
Cods-head with Shrimps.

Second Course.

Roasted Pheasants and Partridges
Bisque of Shel-Fish
Tanzy
Dish of roasted Ducks and Teals
Jole of Sturgeon
Pear Tart Cream'd
Dish of Sweetmeats
Dish of Fruit of Sorts.

BOOKS

BOOKS printed for and sold by Maurice Atkins, *at the* Golden-Ball *in S.* Paul's *Church-Yard.*

FOLIO.

THE great Historical, Geographical, Genealogical, and Poetical Dictionary; Being a curious Miscellany of Sacred and Prophane History. Containing, in short, the Lives and most Remarkable Actions of the Patriarchs, Judges, and Kings of the *Jews*. Of the Apostles, Fathers, and Doctors of the Church. Of Popes, Cardinals, Bishops, *&c.* Collected from the best Historians, Chronologers, and Lexicographers, as *Clavisius*, *Helvicus*, *Isaacson*, *Marsham*, *Baudrand*, *Hoffman*, *Lloyd*, *Chevreau*, and others, but more especially out of *Lewis Morery*, D. D. his Eighth Edition, Corrected and Enlarged by Mons. *Le Clerc.* The Second Edition, Revis'd, Corrected and Enlarged to the Year 1688. By *Jer. Collier*, A. M. and continu'd to this Time by another Hand. In Three Volumes.

The Ecclesiastical History of *Great-Britain*, chiefly of *England*; from the first planting of Christianity, to the end of the Reign of King *Charles* II. with a Brief Account of the Affairs of Religion in *Ireland*. Collected from the best ancient Historians, Councils, and Records By *Jer. Collier*, A. M. In Two Volumes.

Lexicon Technicum; or an Universal *English* Dictionary of Arts and Sciences, Explaining not only the Terms of Art, but the Arts themselves. By *John Harris*, D. D. F R. S. In 2 Vol.

A

A Paraphrase and Annotations upon all the Books of the New Testament; briefly explaining all the difficult Places thereof. The 7th Edit. Corrected and Enlarged, by *H Hammond*, D. D.

The Works of the Right Reverend and Learned *Ezekiel Hopkins*, late Lord Bishop of *London-Derry* in *Ireland*: Collected into one Volume.

Index Villaris; or an exact Register, Alphabetically digested, of all the Cities, Market-Towns, Parishes, Villages, the Hundred, Lath, Rape, Ward, Wapentake, or other Division of each County: The Bishopricks, Deanries, Churches, Chappels, Hospitals, with the Rectories and Vicarages in *England* and *Wales*, and their respective Valuations in the King's Books.

A complete Book of Arithmetick, in Four Books, by *Samuel Jeake*, Merchant.

OCTAVO.

AN Introduction to the History of the principal Kingdoms and States of *Europe*, with an Appendix never printed before; containing an Introduction to the History of the principal Sovereign States of *Italy*, particularly *Venice*, *Modena*, *Mantua*, *Florence*, and *Savoy*. The 6th Edit Corrected and Improv'd. By *Sam. Puffendorf*, Counsellor of State to the late King of *Sweden*.

An Introduction to the History of the principal Kingdoms and States of *Asia*, *Africa*, and *America*, both ancient and modern, according to the Method of *Sam. Puffendorf*, Counsellor of State to the late King of *Sweden*.

Reflexions upon Ridicule, or what it is that makes a Man Ridiculous, and the means to avoid it. Wherein are represented the different Manners and Characters of Persons of the present Age. Of Unpoliteness, Indiscretion, Affectation, foolish Vanity, the bad Taste, Im-

Imposture, the morose Humour, Impertinence: Of Prejudice, Interest, Sufficiency, Absurdities, Caprice, false Delicacy, Decorum.

Reflexions upon the Politeness of Manners, with Maxims for Civil Society. Being the 2d Part of the Reflexions upon Ridicule. By the same Hand. Of Politeness, modest Sentiments, Discretion, *&c.* Moderation, *&c.* Complaisance. Of genteel Behaviour, Sincerity, Maxims for Civil Society.

The History of the *Bucaniers* of *America*, from their first Original, down to this Time. Written in several Languages, and now collected into one Vol. Illustrated with 25 Copper Plates.

A Complete History of *Europe*; or a View of the Affairs thereof, Civil and Military, from the beginning of the Treaty of *Nimeguen*, 1676, to the end of the Year 1700.

A Complete History of the *Turks*, from their Original in the Year 755, to the Year 1701. Containing the Rise, Growth and Decay of that Empire, in its respective Periods, under their several Kings and Emperors. With a new Map of the *Turkish* Empire. Design'd and Engrav'd by Mr. *Moll* In 2 Vol.

Essays upon several moral Subjects, in 4 Parts. Of Pain, Revenge, Authors, Power, Infancy and Youth, Riches and Poverty, Whoredom, Drunkenness, Usury, an Apostle, Solitude. By *Jeremy Collier*, M. A. The Second Edition.

The History of *Lapland*. Containing a Geographical Description, and a Natural History of that Country: With an Account of the Inhabitants, their Original, Religion, Customs, Habits, Marriages, Conjurations, Employments, *&c.* Written by *John Scheffer*.

The wise and ingenious Companion, *French* and *English*: Being a Collection of the Wit of the Illustrious Persons, both ancient and modern. By Mr. *Boyer*, Author of the Royal Dictionary.

The

The Gazetteer; or Newsman's Interpreter, in 2 Parts: Being a Geographical Index of all the considerable Cities, Patriarchships, Bishopricks, Universities, Dukedoms, Earldoms, and such-like, Imperial and Hance-Towns, Ports, Forts, Castles, &c. in the whole World, shewing in what Kingdoms, Provinces, and Counties they are; to what Prince they are now subject. The 9th Edit Corrected and very much Enlarg'd, with the Addition of a Table of the Births, Marriages, &c. of all the Kings, Princes, and Potentates. By *Lawrence Eachard.*

Glossographia Anglicana Nova, or a Dictionary, interpreting such hard Words, of whatever Language, as are at present us'd in the *English* Tongue, with their Etymologies, Definitions, &c. also the Terms of Divinity, Law, Physick, Mathematicks, History, Agriculture, Logick, Metaphysick, Grammar, Poetry, Musick, Heraldry, Architecture, Painting, War, and all other Arts and Sciences are herein explain'd, from the best and modern Authors, as Sir *Isaac Newton*, Dr *Harris*, Dr. *Gregory*, *Mr. Lock*, *Mr. Evelyn*, *Mr. Dryden*, *Mr. Blount*, &c. Very useful to all those that desire to understand what they read.

The Peerage of *England*, or an Historical and Genealogical Account of the Present Nobility. Containing the Descent, Original Creations, and most Remarkable Actions of them, and their respective Ancestors. Also the Chief Titles of Honour and Preferment they now enjoy; with their Marriages and Issue, continu'd to this present Year 1710 Collected as well from our best Historians, publick Records, and other sufficient Authorities, as from the personal Informations of the Nobility To which is prefix'd, an Introduction of the present Royal Family of *Great-Britain*, trac'd thro' its several Branches down to this Time, and terminating with the Protestant Succession. This last Printed for *Abel Roper*, at the *Black-Boy* in *Fleetstreet*.

Lightning Source UK Ltd.
Milton Keynes UK
UKOW041459200212

187624UK00006B/132/P